Author's Note: I didn't write *Eight Billion Steps* as a "How to beat cancer" book; however, it does contain some practical information that may help.

Eight
Billion
Steps:

My Impossible Quest
For Cancer Comedy

ISBN-13: 978-1484835647
ISBN-10: 1484835646

Eight Billion Steps:
My Impossible Quest For Cancer Comedy

by

Jeffrey Penn May

Also by Jeffrey Penn May

Margery

Cynthia and the Blue Cat's Last Meow

No Teacher Left Standing

Where the River Splits

Roobala Take Me Home

Finding Your Fiction:
Concise Steps to Writing Successful Fiction

ACKNOWLEDGMENTS

Thank you to those who saved my life, and enhanced my quality of life, especially my wife, Kim, my family and friends who are hopefully represented favorably in my narrative, and to the healthcare professionals, all of them in this book, including those who may or may not have made a mistake. I am thankful to the doctors, their intellect, hard work, and dedication, especially to those who, knowingly or not, contributed their own peculiar brand of humor, listed here in order of appearance: doctors Andrew Chao, Fredrick Pugliano, Marc Vavares, Hiram Gay, Tonya Wildes, Jason Diaz, Jeffrey Jorgensen, Gregory Weinstein, Michael Kupferman, Brian Nussenbaum, Bruce Haughey, Martin Clarke, Archie Harmon. And to the following organizations, SSM St. Clare Health Center, Saint Louis University Hospital, University of Missouri Hospital, MD Anderson Cancer Center, University of Pennsylvania Hospital, Siteman Cancer Center, and Barnes-Jewish Hospital. To all the therapists, specifically Shannon Nana and Shelly Ryan, and nurses, especially the ones at Barnes.

For the 2023 Update, thank you to those who persevered through the Covid pandemic and continued to provide high quality care, specifically those who contributed to, like those before them, often elusive humor. Thank you to Jane and Jerry at St. Luke hyperbaric wound care center, Doctor Ryan Jackson, Melissa Portell and Lisa Shoemaker, Doctor James Boyd, therapists Kaitlen Keister and Kacie Brooks, and from Mercy Integrative medicine Jenny, Jen, and Shannon.

Table of Contents

Introduction

This book was going to be *Two Hundred Steps, My Fight Against Cancer*, but the title seemed too generic for what was percolating in my sometimes painfully clear mind. So I changed it from the typical to the absurd, and I have been struggling with my quest ever since.

Still, the initial inspiration might be worth noting. The number two hundred referred to counting steps – wheeling an IV pole from my hospital room down the stark gray-carpeted hallway, through the waiting area and past elevators and restroom, and then left down a windowless, narrow hallway, about enough room for a wheelchair, with brilliantly shiny wood floors. My IV wheels hummed on that floor. I loved that floor. As much as any captive animal might love pacing in its cage. I turned around at what was for me a dead end because there wasn't much sense trying to escape an inescapable reality and bash my pole through a steel door to crash down the stairway. Eventually, I'd take the elevator. I counted the steps back to my room. Two hundred. More or less.

Along the way I noticed "exciting things." The fire hose. The office doors. The floor. Interesting people. A thin woman with glasses admiring the perfect floor then pushing hard on the stairwell door. I wanted to reassure her. But then I realized she was looking down only to avoid looking at me.

A middle aged woman wheeling boxes of soda-pop and chemically laden snacks, and I thought: How can anyone remotely associated with health and healing consume such crap? Then there was the closet marked "air tanks." And from this dubious launching point, I will tell you that going on a "quest for cancer comedy" isn't going to be easy. For example, they could have opened that closest for me and "for the rest of my life," I could be wheeling around scuba gear.

So, as far as I can tell, there has been almost nothing humorous about the whole trip, other than the strange, weird, odd kind of funny. Nothing that would suggest comedy. But I'm making the effort, attempting it because I have a habit of setting expectations so high, and falling so short, the fall sometimes elicits a chuckle.

As I write this, I see that I've already screwed up – I must fully believe in a "full recovery" or I will have no chance at "full recovery." But if I know that I always set unrealistically high expectations only to fall short, then how can I truly believe in full recovery? See how "funny" it can get?

Before... what a cliché, but as I would learn through this ordeal, clichés are remarkably true. Before... I would avoid any book about illness, especially cancer. Bookstores were troublesome. If I wandered down the wrong aisle and saw a bunch of cancer books, I'd look away as if I'd accidentally stared at the sun. I hid my psyche just like the little kids hiding behind moms and dads when they saw me walking through the hospital pushing my IV-pole, dripping bags, grizzly white beard sticking through bandages, tube up my nose. The little ones clung to their parents, stared at me with wide eyes, and glanced back to make sure I wasn't following them. My wife, Kim, laughed when she saw this. "The little dudes," she said. "They think you're really scary."

With very little evidence other than my own harrowing experience, I have come to the conclusion that cancer stories follow a well-worn pattern of disbelief, denial, acceptance, treatment, and so on, depending on the final outcome, and they're usually not funny. Not that cancer comedy hasn't been tried. In 2011, a movie based on a true cancer story was about "finding humor in unlikely places" with a "stoner twist." I avoided seeing that movie for the same reasons I avoid books about cancer, and skimming the plot synopsis just confirmed my decision.

So why read this book? Because it's a comedy of course. It's damn funny. A hilarious, best-in-the-world joke. You're going to fall on the floor laughing. Where's my lampshade?

Why did I change my number to Eight Billion? Because sometime after having counted up to two hundred for what felt like two hundred times, I blurted out in the long narrow hallway, "Screw the damn steps!" My speech was muffled because of the tight bandages, and because I was choking back thick, proliferating thrush-crud. I'm sure that when the janitor looked at me and smiled, he'd heard only unintelligible garble.

So I abandoned my original number and chose eight because it's my favorite number. Turned on its side, it's the symbol for infinity, and if you let your mind go there, infinity looks a lot like hell. A "billion" because a "million" isn't what it used to be, and it's also a movie reference and everything is always a reference to something else because there is "nothing new under the sun," which is, if you think about it and read the entire bible passage, particularly depressing. Reminds me of a Beatles song lyric, "nothings going to change my world."

Even now, writing this paragraph in a respite between my third surgery and radiation, I haven't found myself wanting to read any books about cancer. Even Lance Armstrong's *It's Not About the Bike*. I tried. But his early discussion about all those who died and his musings about why he was spared put my mind in a bad place. I would have preferred reading about the bike. Or more about his drugs, "recovering" his way to all those Tour de France titles. I want some of those drugs. Only to cheat death of course. Not win a bicycle race.

Maybe I am changing; maybe I will find the courage to read cancer tales someday. But is it even a matter of courage? Or just my way of dealing with it? Avoidance is not the same as denial. Avoiding details about my treatment is a technique.

I deny that my avoidance is denial!

At least let's make a distinction between the two. And accept that there is a place for denial as well. Denying cancer is a way to fight it. I may have it, but it stops here and now. It cannot exist; therefore, it will not. Of course, avoidance and denial have their limitations. So, my mental gymnastics involved acceptance, followed by avoidance and denial, followed by acceptance, and so on.

I walk a tightrope, needing to know and not wanting to know. For example, one radiologist was going to give me his spiel about "what to expect" from high doses of radiation. I said, "No thanks." I already knew it wasn't going to be fun, that it was, in fact, going to be downright awful. No sense dwelling on the particulars. Instead, I thought, I am going to have as much fun as possible learning to swallow prior to radiation so that I can lose that function during radiation and relearn it after. It is that sort of convoluted logic that sustains me. Only the essential information please. Half hour or so five days a week, ten minutes of actual radiation time. That's it. Don't want to know about the skin burns, the scorched throat, muscles turning rubbery, like chicken too long in the microwave... see? Who wants to think about that?

Survivor stories are great but spare me the horrific details. Don't even use the word "horrific." Fortunately, I have a brilliant wife who saved my life, researching all the ghastly details, allowing me to focus on the positive and compartmentalize my terror to doctor visits and surgery.

In an April 12, 2012 email to family and close friends, I think I was clear enough in my request for help. I needed them to believe, to tell me I was going to be "just fine." I updated them about my "situation," telling them that after lots of travel, research, and consternation, my wife Kim and I decided we would move to Houston for about three months, that we would have surgery and radiation at MD Anderson.

A few days later, everything changed dramatically. I actually used the word "dramatic" in a text message. It's the only time that I can recall ever using that word and meaning it. Dramatic!

My descriptions of what happened are going to be false. But in essence they are true. It's just impossible for me to give a wholly accurate description. And a lot will be second hand info. I'll do my best, though. And Kim has her own story. If she ever chooses to write it, I'm sure it will be "interesting" especially compared to my account.

Generally this book is being written in 2012, many drafts written during the process, and during recovery. Right now it's May 22. However, on May 24, I will have another surgery, and it will knock me on my ass, and I will become a little down about the whole thing. And I will get a text message from my friend Julie, "You'll be fine Jeff:)"

Chapter One - Life is Good!

I ran two miles in the morning, hiked five miles, and biked seven in the evening. In between, I mowed the lawn, cleaned the kitchen, made love with my wife, and wrote a short story. Not every day of course and I confess to hyperbole, but you get the idea. Even though I complained about real and imaginary aches and pains, at 58 I was in great shape, and was eating healthily, more or less vegetarian, with lots of natural micro-nutrients. I waded clear Missouri Ozark streams casting my fly rod into deep pools and catching brilliant multicolored sunfish and gloriously aggressive smallmouth bass. After admiring my catch, I released the fish back into the cool current. Occasionally, I'd sit on the stream bank and smoke a cigar. Sometimes, while fishing with my brothers, I drank too much. My brother Jim called it "over-beverage-ing."

Of course, it wasn't all good. My childhood dream of making a "living" by writing fiction had disintegrated. At some point, our dreams become delusions and we set new expectations for ourselves. However, because I had lots of "close calls" with big publishing houses, I held onto my dreams far too long, far past the point when I should have given up and pursued professorship or shifted to selling books or lampshades or classy underwear. Or I could have been a financier! Then I'd be loaded with money and happiness and... would that have prevented my cancer?

In the early 1980's Scribners responded to my first novel: "Many moments are beautiful, witty, and surprising, and I was beguiled by many aspects of *Roobala*." I didn't pin all my hopes on one novel of course. But I never gave up on *Roobala*. In 2011, I completed the last of twenty rewrites of

Roobala Take Me Home a first and forever masterpiece (even if only in my own mind).

Mercifully, however, I lost faith, even though I've won awards (hasn't everyone), was nominated for a Pushcart Prize (apparently not as weighty as it once was), and *Where the River Splits* was published by a small company that succumbed to the Great Recession just as the novel received an exceptional review in the St. Louis Post-Dispatch. I'd also published poetry, short stories, and articles. But measured against the time, ink and paper, and rejections, my so-called accomplishments were the equivalent of dying at the base of a glacier, still 10,000 feet from the summit, leaving me teaching English Composition at a technical college, and getting paid part-time wages for full-time work. After some angst, in which I felt like an actor in a tacky "tortured artist" movie, I accepted my fate. My "writing career," such as it was, sucked. But, by God, I was healthy! Oh, I'd still write of course, but now armed with the knowledge that I'd made too many bad decisions based on delusions, I envisioned writing nonfiction with uplifting titles such as *Confessions of a Failed Novelist*.

Meanwhile, in the geologic milliseconds before the recession, Kim and I sent her sister Anne, and her husband John, a huge check, a short bridge loan into an abyss. John's Denver spec house, which would have sold for two million, steadily became worthless, or at least less than he owed, and he owed us 65,000, a line-of-credit on our own home. Not to worry though because he was paying the interest on the loan. But as John lost one property after another, he stopped payments, and twenty years of sweat equity went flapping about in the wind. I could see the prayer flag on some distant mountaintop with the truism in bright red letters – never lend money to relatives.

Our 21 year old son, Sam, and 19 year old daughter, Sarah, were living at home and trying to figure out what to do with their lives, the former a landscaper, the latter a Barista at Starbucks. Eventually, they'll want to go back to college. Like many of you, paying for college seems out of reach. What savings we have left depend on which way the financial wind blows, and it blows a lot.

My parents lived alone, independently, in Belleville, Illinois, almost an hour's drive and, at 92 and 93, their health was becoming problematic. My Dad already had two hip replacements and one shattered hip repair, and my Mom was repeating herself, repeating herself after only a minute or two. Kim's parents were 82 and 83. Her mom had spent a year in and out of hospitals near death only to miraculously stabilize. Her dad doesn't see very well and her mom can't remember much. On the way to one medical appointment, he blindly took the wheel while she told him where to turn. They got there eventually.

Kim was an outstanding elementary school teacher suffering the cruelty of a principal with narcissistic personality disorder. (Either that or she was a psychopath, but I always like to think the best of people). In 2007, while blaming Kim for disrupting the first-grade team, the principal grabbed her and screamed, "I'm your boss!" The teacher responsible for the chaos turned out to have severe mental disorders. In May 2011, the "boss" launched another twisted verbal attack, shifted blame, and wrote a false evaluation with impossible job targets. The teacher's union helped amend the evaluation and the boss agreed based on the assumption that Kim was going to retire.

We planned a trip to Hawaii. We had visited every other state. Including Alaska. So our island paradise waited for us.

Chapter Two – A Bump, Not A Lump

Sometime in the Fall of 2011, a bump appeared on the right side of my neck, noticeable probably because I was eating more or less according to Joel Fuhrman's *Eat to Live* and I had lost ten pounds, on purpose. I started fiddling with my bump, pushing on it, squeezing it. Curious, I thought, that it got bigger because of my fiddling. I put ice packs on it. That would fix it. My wife said, "Don't worry about it, it's probably just cancer."

We all complain about minor health issues, but at times I've unnecessarily freaked out over them, making them worse. If you panic, minor health issues can subject you to surgery, occasionally at the hands of some hack. But I responded to this particular bump with astonishing aplomb. It didn't hurt. Nothing seemed wrong. I had plenty of other things to worry about. This bump was nothing but a bump.

November 1, 2011 my son Sam and I went to our family doctor, Andrew Chao, for a routine office visit, and I offhandedly suggested that I had a bump on my neck. But I added quickly, "It's always been there." Always, I guess, is a relative term.

My "right side" always had problems. My one rotting wisdom tooth was on the right side, and a few years ago I had it removed. After it's removal, I drooled. My wife and kids mocked me for slurping like a drooling old man, so I taught myself not to slurp or at least to hide it when I did. Then a crown on the molar wouldn't stay on and eventually that tooth had to be removed. I asked both the oral surgeon and the dentist what the drool was all about. The dentist said that it was a reaction to the missing molar, and the oral surgeon said, "Beats the hell out of me." Neither of them noticed that my tongue was crooked.

After my casual mention about the bump that had always been there, my son said, "I never noticed it before."

Doctor Chao felt it and said, "I've never felt that before."

And soon, November 8, 2011, I was getting an ultrasound at a shiny new hospital called Saint Clare in Fenton, about 10 minutes from our home. I was in and out promptly, no reason for alarm, nice place, and gee, what was the big deal really? It was sure to be nothing more that a cyst of some sort. Hardly noticeable. Didn't hurt. Once confirmed benign, I could choose to have it removed or not.

Even with that sort of confidence, phone calls about test results are great fun, aren't they? You see the caller ID. You instinctively know it's the doctor even if you don't recognize the number or it's restricted. The surge of adrenaline starts before you answer. The jolt makes your day memorable. Likely, people have the same sort of jolt when told they've inherited a million dollars. This phone call was just the flip side. Someone tossed a coin, I called heads, and got the unfortunate tail.

Doctor Chao called while I was driving home from an errand, and told me, with some urgency, that I needed to see an "ear-nose-throat guy" because "we don't know what it is."

"But," I said, "it's nothing to worry about, right?"

He avoided agreeing with me by repeating "we don't know what it is" and that I needed to see "an ear-nose-throat guy." After my initial adrenaline surge, his ambiguous response didn't bother me much. It was nothing. It didn't hurt.

The next day, we got our Hawaii vacation confirmation for Poipu Beach, Koloa. We were going to Hawaii on the cheap, using credit card points for the flight, using my father-in-law's time-share for the resort, and staying several days with my Aunt and cousins who live in Hilo. Planning the trip was a welcome distraction from my bump.

On November 17, I went to Saint Clare and the ENT guy Doctor Fredrick Pugliano. He was a geek, awkward with patients, standing as if always holding an imaginary clipboard, balding in the back, and an even voice with an erratic delivery. I sort of liked him, despite his habit of repeating my name "Mr. May." Once I asked him to call me Jeff, but he said that because he was "so much younger," he had trouble calling me by my first name. He couldn't have been that much younger. I was only 58. Come on, this guy had to be in his forties.

While waiting for Doctor Fred and his assistant to stick a long biopsy needle into my neck, I told them about one doctor who had his finger fully up my rectum when he casually said, "So, have any other of your family members had prostate cancer?" I think the assistant laughed. Maybe Doctor Fred smiled and made a short "huh" noise. A good sign?

Doctor Fred slowly inserted the long the needle into my neck, surprisingly painless, and withdrew it, then placed the fluids on a slide and said, "Interesting."

"Interesting?" I said.

In disturbing contrast to their previous reaction, they fell silent, staring at the sample, preparing it for testing, then the assistant suggested a follow-up visit for Tuesday, November 22.

I declined quickly. I'm not a numerologist, but I wanted to avoid November 22; it seemed weighted with too much historical and personal significance, the birth and death of my firstborn, events I wrote about in "The Wells Creek Route." (The Pushcart recognition, while satisfying, didn't make the initial experience any less painful.)

Doctor Fred was going out of town, a technique all doctors seem to use after serious office visits, never mind that it was Thanksgiving. But I was reasonable. I recognized that this guy just might have a family, although I didn't see them sitting around a big table laughing about cancer. So the next appointment would have to be November 28, at which time I was to get another ultrasound, with contrast, requiring an IV.

I responded to this wait as anyone might, going about my life normally. With my bump. I put ice on it, but otherwise ignored it and slogged through Thanksgiving, driving to Belleville with mashed potatoes, green beans, and Turkey breast, taking the "moveable feast" to my parents. Then on to a large family gathering at Kim's other sister's, Beth Ketcher and her husband Brad.

And of course, we did what most teachers do on holidays – graded papers.

Monday the 28th I drove from my job at the technical college near downtown St. Louis, to Fenton, rushed in and got my ultrasound with contrast, waited for the results on CD, took the elevator upstairs, and arrived at the doctor's office promptly, feeling good about my punctuality, and my responsible use of time.

Cheerily, I skipped into Doctor Fred's office, with my CD which would show him the easy options, fully expecting to hear it was a benign bump. ("Benign bump" had the added advantage of being alliterative. I still have trouble with "cancer comedy.") We could remove it, or just leave it alone. Peering through his glasses, standing near his office door, Doctor Fred said, "Mr. May, the lab report shows a low grade mucoepidermoid carcinoma."

"Say what?"

"It's extremely rare."

He said something else but I'll be damned if I know what it was. I recovered from the emotional blow and suddenly possessed laser-like focus. I asked pointed questions. Typical questions likely being repeated across the globe at this moment. "Yes," Doctor Fred answered, "I trust the lab. No, no reason to take another biopsy."

"This isn't," I said, "what I expected."

"Me neither."

But he must have been suspicious. When he said "interesting" that meant it was interesting for a reason, right? I've used "interesting" for all sorts of things. Like when I put a fishhook through my calf and had to sit down and start carving it out with a dull knife. Fortunately, my brother John waded up with his sharp knife and performed streamside surgery with alacrity. Or when my brother Jim and I were trying to get the window to my old Dodge Grand Caravan up, because the small electric motor wasn't working, and he pulled with needle nose pliers while I pushed the up button and the window exploded in the door. That was interesting.

"What happens if I just leave it in?"

"Well Mr. May, you don't want to go around with a cancerous lump in your neck. You will want to get it out."

"So it's low grade?"

"Yes."

"And that's better than high-grade?"

"Yes."

"Great!" I said, "I'll take low-grade!"

He remained humorless, leaning against the wall, arms across his chest, more verification of what I was up against. What sort of joke was this?

Sensing that I might ask another question, Doctor Fred eased open his office door and leaned out like a robot in a hurry. He's a good guy. Just not too good on patient interaction. I asked for the pathology report and felt a little better reading "low-grade" in print. And even better when I read it was only "suspicious" of low-grade. Other things couldn't be ruled out. Those other things weren't necessarily cancer. Or at least I didn't think they were as I read it over and over again.

Other neoplasms or reactive entities,
such as chronic sialoadenitis
with abundant metaplasia,
are not entirely excluded.

That didn't sound like cancer to me. More like sixteenth century poetry. I had to read it repeatedly to make any sense of it. And my bump didn't hurt, so it was nothing. Remember, I thought, to take what doctors say with a grain of salt, my life turning into a cancer cliché. As an English Composition instructor, the clichés were troubling.

I couldn't think of anything else to say, and clearly the doctor and his staff were ready to go, so I left. I must have sounded shaky when I called Kim.

"Do you want me to come get you," she asked.

I avoided researching mucoepidermoid carcinoma because I shared things in common with the nineteenth century writer Jerome K. Jerome. In the opening scene of his classic semi-autobiographical comic novel *Three Men In Boat*, he is looking for a hay fever treatment and casually begins reading about other diseases. By the time he's finished, he concludes that he has every disease on the list. "I had walked into that reading-room a happy healthy man. I crawled out a decrepit wreck."

In the 21st century, symptoms, ailments, and treatments have expanded exponentially, and a few clicks online can elicit total body panic, usually in the middle of the night. Even when I try to avoid cyber induced illnesses, I'm confronted with TV ads reminding me that I pee too frequently or I should be getting more frequent and longer lasting erections. Doctors then dole out pharmaceutical samples, orders tests, and send me on my way more convinced than ever that my few remaining days on earth will be "quite miserable." Are writers prone to this sort of panic?

Doctor Fred's assistant suggested I schedule the surgery before the holidays, but when I called the official scheduler, the earliest available date was January 9, 2012. I was tempted to blow it all off as merely a doctor driven surgery, completely unnecessary for a simple little bump.

December was fun, finishing the semester, meeting with friends and family, drinking beer and peeing from the deck at night when Kim wasn't looking, and ignoring my bump, now apparently a "lump," as if it were going to be nothing more than cosmetic surgery. I was lucky to have a home that backed up to woods, lucky to have a family and friends. Life was good. The lump didn't worry me at all. I absolutely knew that it was nothing. It didn't hurt.

I felt pretty good about myself. I'd gotten over my troubled artist crisis. I'd accepted that I was a failure in areas where I'd set impossibly high standards. But I was more or less successful in being married and raising two kids who were kind, considerate, hard working, helpful, and articulate. And we had potential college money in savings and equity. Except the $65,000.

I was fine. I'd only be in the hospital overnight, and then

I could go back to work. I'd miss only the first day of the semester. Go in, get the lump removed, and move on with my life, tackle all the problems, help Kim with her retirement, help the kids with finding themselves, write articles and book reviews. Maybe even try to promote my books. Had I paid closer attention to the details, I might have known that I was going to have a "neck dissection." Based on the term alone, I might have known I couldn't go back to work for a week. I'd been teaching at the technical college for over seven years and never missed a day. But as a contractual employee, I didn't get sick days. If I didn't show up, I didn't get paid. But at least I had a job.

Chapter Three –
Just A Little Neck Dissection

Anyone who has had significant surgery knows that the surgery itself is not much to the patient. After all, we're out cold. The anesthesia works great, much better than whiskey. On the other hand, sometimes whiskey will do. If I was sprawled in the sagebrush with a bullet in my neck and my grinning demented pal pulled out his big knife stained from gutting last night's deer, I would gladly guzzle whiskey. However, if time travel were possible, I would eschew the past and embrace the future, hoping that medicine and technology would continue its advance, and tumors would be removed easily and painlessly by scientific magic. Not dirty knives.

When I emerged from the surgery haze, I was sitting in a barbershop like chair. Only in retrospect did it seem a little odd. Normally, I meditate while sitting, so that's what I did, repeating my mantra and slipping off into a comforting calm self-awareness far from the reality of hospitals. Apparently, this set off alarms. And alarmed the attending nurses. They pumped me with oxygen. I heard my wife explain that I was probably just meditating. Once the oxygen forced me awake, I consciously remained in the reality of the moment. I didn't want to startle anyone, and I did not like the beeping. Soon I was being wheeled back to my spacious, comfortable private room, designed by patients, nurses, doctors, and architects, complete with refrigerator, space for a wheelchair, couch for visitors. Nice pad if you were single.

Everything was fine. I had a drainage tube sticking out from my neck, but I didn't feel too bad, and I ordered a fruit plate for dinner. No big deal.

Kim and my daughter Sarah chatted with me and everything was just fine, there was nothing wrong, the dissection went well. It would be a few days before we got the pathology report. I believed that Doctor Fred removed all the cancer and I was home free. Before leaving, Kim suggested I call Sam, let him know I was okay. He had avoided the hospital, and I didn't blame him. At his age, I would have done the same thing.

"Hey buddy," I said, "how's it going?"

"Okay..."

"What?" I asked.

"Nothing, it's just..."

"Just what?"

"Just that if it were me," he said, "I'd want to know, that's all."

"Know what?"

"You need to know eventually. I don't understand why you don't just face up to it now."

"Let me talk to your mother."

Kim explained what I didn't want to hear. She and Sarah had talked to Doctor Fred after the surgery. An awkward conversation in which Doctor Fred kept repeating that he couldn't believe how big the tumor was, much bigger than he expected, and they had to take out the jugular vein because the tumor was wrapped around it. (Who knew we have more than one jugular?) And they needed to do more tests.

"I'm so sorry, honey, but you said you didn't want to know."

Apparently, I had already implemented my avoidance technique, and during December while I was so productively drinking beer and pissing from the deck, Kim researched mucoepidermoid carcinoma. Of course I had avoided using the "C" word. I used "tumor" freely, but saying the C-word was an acknowledgement that I was in deep trouble. I was, of course. But I wasn't anywhere near ready to accept it. One afternoon while Kim was driving us home from one of what would be a gazillion trips to the pharmacy, I was on the phone with my brother Jim in Wyoming, using words such as "bump" and "thing" (of all things), and Kim suggested I tell him that I had cancer. I held my hand up, palm against her, and said, "Don't say that word!" I was trying to control my destiny by avoiding the obvious reality. On the phone, Jim laughed, understanding the implications, because he was often besieged by signs and omens and knows the power of words.

I could hardly be upset with Kim for not telling me, for doing exactly what I wanted. In fact, I felt a twinge of guilt because it was a burden she would have to bear throughout the process, having to decide when and where to tell me things, and when to withhold information. She didn't always get it right, but she came close to perfection, a skill I'm still trying to figure out. I am in awe of her. I don't know how she did it.

Sam got back on the phone, and I told him that I wished he hadn't said anything, explaining that not knowing would have allowed me at least one more evening, one more night, believing that everything would be okay.

"Now I feel really bad," he said.

What kind of jerk was I? I was laying guilt on him. "Don't worry about it. You're right. I would have to know eventually."

"Do you want me to come over?"

"Sure, buddy, come over for awhile. I'd love to see you."

Fifteen minutes later, he was sitting across from me as I lay in the hospital bed, struggling for some humor. "Nice place, huh."

"Yeah," he said.

"It's like a hotel room."

When he was a kid, as I tucked him in at night, I'd always ask, "Do you have any questions?" Mostly, he didn't, but when he did, they were important questions.

"What to you think is going to happen?" he asked.

At a time when I needed to conjure up Yoda, or at least recall *Zen and the Art of Motorcycle Maintenance*, I responded with the worst case scenario, precisely what I wanted to avoid. I don't know if it was the right response or not. Of course, if Sam ever reads this, he'll likely have a different interpretation. But my logic seemed sound. I wanted him to acknowledge his emotions, thinking that like most young men, he bottles them up and eventually they'd take their toll.

"I think," I said, "I'm going to suffer a slow and painful death."

"Yeah," he said, "me too."

That did it. We hugged, and he cried. So I suppose my approach worked. Except that it ran counter to my coping strategy, and my words ring clear today, bubbling into my reality, annoying the hell out of me, having to subdue them, the expectation of suffering and death. I will have a full recovery! And, by the way, I will make it funny! (So far, my failure seems obvious.)

After Sam left, I lay in that hospital bed unwilling to sleep. It was the first time I'd spent the night in the hospital since I was four with pneumonia, under an oxygen tent, and a nurse gave me a plastic yellow race car, one of my earliest memories, along with seeing the movie *One Hundred and One Dalmatians*, a number, by the way, that pales next to my eight billion.

I sent a text message to Kim.

Sarah texted back, "Mom is getting some good sleep. Can you talk to me instead?"

"Tomorrow makes me sad."

"Well that's silly," Sarah responded, "Why are you sad about tomorrow?"

I've lost my text message reply. It has disappeared into the electronic netherworld. Piecing together what happened is difficult, but without documentation, how is anyone supposed to get it even close to right? Our memories cloud things enough as it is. But I'm fairly sure I was sad because I knew I would have to face the harsh realities of what lie ahead, and what lie ahead was much worse than what I was thinking at the time.

In the morning, I climbed out of bed and paced around the room. I was finished with this hospital stay. I had a slash across my neck, a drainage tube leading to the pocket of my hospital gown and a squeeze-toy container filled with frothy pinkish fluids, which reminded me of "precious bodily fluids" from Stanley Kubrick's *Doctor Strangelove*, a movie I'd seen at least six times and wanted to forget. I paced, not very stealthily, but like a zoo animal nonetheless. It was obvious that I no longer needed to be there, even though I was told that the "normal" stay after such a procedure is about three days.

I spent only one night in the hospital. I know that statement smacks of boasting, but I need to believe in my resiliency, strength, and resolve. It's entirely likely that I was being a self-centered idiot, but when you're trying to survive, it's sometimes useful to be self-centered. (I'm not sure if it is ever useful to be an idiot.) Here's a little more boasting: A day after surgery, on January 10, I sent lucid emails to my boss about returning to work. I can prove it because I still have the emails. And on January 15, we got another email about our Hawaii vacation. Before too long we would be strolling down a beach near Hilo with my cousins and my aunt, then flying to the resort on Kauai.

Within a week, I was running again. I felt fine. I sent a text message to a friend, "First run, no falls." My strength was good. The tumor was so big it intimidated Doctor Fred, but I had convinced myself that he had gotten it all out and I was fine. Just fine. I felt good. Sure, the left side of my lip made my smile a bit crooked, and when I shaved, it felt strange because the nerves had been sliced and I knew that it would take some time before they regenerated. But I was getting there. Belief in a full recovery helps the neurotransmitters form new pathways. Nerves can regenerate even at 58. I went back to work teaching English Composition, and other than having to work a little harder at enunciating my words, no problem.

Chapter Four –
Phone Calls from Doctor Fred

Doctor Fred called me. If he is awkward in person, you can imagine what he was like on the phone. He said, "Mr. May, we need to schedule a PET scan for you." After that, his abrupt silence was startling. I recovered enough to ask the obvious "why" question. "We need to find the primary source of the tumor."

After a tortured conversation, I figured out that initially he thought the low-grade carcinoma was coming from a gland in the neck, but he didn't find any cancerous salivary glands. Only the one lymph node wrapped around my jugular had the big C cells. In my limited understanding, lymph nodes are just filters of some sort, and rarely if ever, the source. Therefore, it had to be coming from somewhere else in my body. Probably in the head and neck area, but it could be, possibly, anywhere. Anywhere? Lung? Brain? Pancreas? If the pancreas, I was doomed. My mind raced. I wasn't prepared for this phone call. However, I was *not* going on the Internet to study lymph nodes. I need only the information that I need to know. (Now I was Yoda sounding like.)

Doctor Fred wanted to schedule a follow-up appointment, and I suggested that there was "no need for that." We'd get the PET scan and he could just call me with the results. "Well Mr. May," he responded, "we'll have a lot to talk about."

What the hell did that mean? In the flurry of phone calls after talking to Doctor Fred, I called my brother Jim, and he reminded me that doctors don't realize the impact of their words and "they say the strangest things."

According to a happy-to-help cancer coordinator, the first available scan date would be in three weeks. Kim, surrounded by inquisitive third-graders, said that the three-week wait for a PET scan was unacceptable. "That's all they had," I said.

Despite the enormous pressure my wife felt trying to teach her little ones while under the scrutiny of a vindictive boss, she was cheerily insistent with a lackadaisical aide in Doctor Fred's office, and rescheduled the scan for that Thursday, January 19.

While Kim, her sister Beth, and Sarah waited, a guy in jeans and knit shirt took me through hallways to where the PET scan truck had docked, connecting to Saint Clare hospital. I felt like an astronaut as we rode a hydraulic lift up to the control room where several technicians sat around monitors. The big PET machine looked like a capsule ready to be positioned on the rocket. Space awaited, but the idea of exploring my "final frontier" quickly lost its luster as I pondered the implications. I was ushered into a closet, and hooked to an IV, fluids flowing cold. I sat and waited, separated by a threadbare curtain from an older lady. At least she looked "older." Maybe she'd merely had a hard life. In front of me was a lightened plastic photo of a waterfall (presumably on Earth). They placed a warm blanket over me and told me not to move, to sit still for forty-five minutes. That wasn't too difficult, as I've meditated that long many times before, and astronauts are known for remaining cool under dire circumstances.

When the technicians came to get the "old" woman, I was roused by the curtain rattling, as if stepping out of a shower, and I watched her being led away to the big machine. I stared at the plastic waterfall for comfort. Nice waterfall, I thought, then drifted off again into my inner space.

A PET scan opening is much less claustrophobic than an MRI. And I liked the casual approach of the technician. I didn't have to undress and put on a gown. All I needed to do was rid myself of metal and since I don't wear metal, all I had to do was push down my belt buckle while lying on my back. They covered me with another warm blanket. And the painless relatively quiet whirring began. However, near the end of the scan, my nose itched, and I had to go to the bathroom. I didn't have a spacesuit to pee in like Alan Shepard in his tiny capsule perched atop the Mercury-Redstone rocket.

But it was over soon enough and I was released to pee and scratch and tell everyone that it was a breeze really, nothing to it, that I'd blasted off to a planet full of old ladies and waterfalls and returned unscathed.

The "lots to talk about" doctor appointment was Friday at the end of the day. I didn't want to go. I argued the point logically. "If I'm going to get bad news," I said, "I don't want to be in some strange office. I want to be home." My argument was flawless I thought. What's to talk about if the PET scan showed cancer rampant throughout my body, as rampant as my thoughts, traveling to every organ, every muscle twitch, and every hint of indigestion symptomatic of death. I imagined all those scenes in movies, the doctor sitting at his big desk, hands folded, the husband and wife sitting across from him in comfortable chairs, the big news revealed right away, and the anguished looks on the actors' faces. But this was no act.

Eventually, I succumbed to the counter argument, which I still don't understand, something about asking questions face to face, and so on. Maybe I knew that with Doctor Fred an office visit was just as awkward as a telephone call, and looking him in the eye would reveal only tentativeness and ambiguity.

We drove to one of Doctor Fred's office locations, not the fifteen minutes to the hospital, but twenty-five minutes south to a strip mall along a busy secondary highway. Kim suggested a Xanax. I didn't want to start popping pills. I've always been sensitive to medications. On the other hand, if a pill made all this go away....

The receptionist causally mentioned that she tried calling to see if we could arrive earlier, as if implying she knew that we had "lots to talk about," and needed even more time than originally scheduled. The wait seemed excruciatingly long until the Xanax kicked in. Eventually, we were called into the examining room. When Doctor Fred arrived, we exchanged pleasantries and shook hands. He stood, flipping through papers.

"So," I said, "How long do I have?"

If I could just get Doctor Fred to laugh, then I'd know everything would be all right.

"It's not that bad, Mr. May."

"See," Kim said, "I told you."

Doctor Fred explained that the technicians report indicated the primary source appeared to be on the floor of the mouth. Eventually, a murky picture emerged. There was some "activity" around the jaw but that appeared to be a refraction from dental work, and it would be a relatively simple surgery to remove the floor-of-mouth tumor. Likely, we could use the same incision location.

"No big deal, right," I said, "cows get hoof and mouth all the time."

I understand that it was a lame joke, but he didn't even try to crack a smile. He asked me to sit in the dentist-like examining chair.

He stuck his rubber gloved hand into my mouth and probed around under my tongue, on the floor of the mouth. "Hmm," he said, then went to his computer, pulled up a copy of the PET scan, and studied it. "I'm going to talk to the lab technician and get back to you."

"What?"

"It's nothing, Mr. May, I just want to make sure that we're both reading this correctly."

"But it's on the floor of my mouth, right, and I'm going to be okay."

He stared at the computer screen, his silence disturbing.

Kim asked, "So the floor of the mouth is an easy surgery?"

"Yes, it is. Everything is generally good news. I just want to be sure."

Then he made his move toward the door. I'd seen this before. Our "we have a lot to talk about" meeting was over in fifteen minutes. It was Friday after all and we were obviously the last appointment of the day, so I understood. They had tried calling to get us in earlier. Had nothing to do with me or any sort of misdiagnosis. But subconsciously, I knew better. Having already listened to him tell me low-grade in the neck, now shifting to the mouth, I suspected worse to come. However, in my attempt to affect the outcome with optimism, I chose to believe the best, that it was simple floor-of-mouth disease; it would require a hospital stay not any more difficult than last time. Mucoepidermoid carcinoma, while rare, had a "high cure rate."

As we were leaving, I congratulated him on doing a fine job with the surgery, knowing of course that surgeons usually have big egos, and feeding his ego might make him do a better job. Sort of like the Navy test pilots I used to work with, except that I rarely felt obliged to compliment them. They knew they were the best of the best and would have viewed a compliment as questioning their skill. They were too good to need compliments. That was in the early 1980s when I worked for McDonnell Aircraft, and was assigned to Pautexent River Naval Air Station. I was a long-haired college graduate with a degree in English and Psychology, and I was testing the maintenance manuals for the Navy's first F-18s. My job was negligible compared to theirs. The pilots had to actually fly the jets. If their split second decisions were wrong, they could lose their lives in a fiery crash. Although bad maintenance manuals could theoretically also cause a crash, I was only one of thousands of people involved, a shared responsibility with purposefully redundant back-ups. I knew my status then, and I knew it with surgeons. I was an English Composition Teacher at a technical college. They were top-notch surgeons.

On Tuesday, January 24, I got an "interesting" phone call from Doctor Fred.

"Ah, Mr. May?"

"Yes."

"We need to schedule you for a biopsy right away."

"Why?"

"It appears that you have a large tumor on the back of

the tongue and throat, possibly more, but we can't tell for sure until we get a biopsy."

I was standing in my office at home. The news, obviously, was significantly more grave than he'd led us to believe.

"Are you okay, Mr. May."

No, I wasn't. But I calmly thanked him and got off the phone.

Prior to this moment, I had shed a tear or two, but recovered quickly, even though often on the verge of panic. This news, however, was more than I could bear. Time warped. No time to put on a smiley face. No time to think about the pile of putty you become, the mess you must look like in front of your daughter, no time to think about your career, your hopes, dreams. You just react. Robert E. Lee wept while apologizing to his men after Picket's charge. My father admitted to crying during WWII. I'm not suggesting that I'm anything like my father who heroically fought his way through Europe, and sometimes survived by pure luck, artillery shell landing at his feet – thump! – and failing to detonate, my father who witnessed his buddies not so fortunate, the sudden tragic severing of limbs and guts spilling out. But we do speak in battle terms – fighting cancer, beating cancer, surviving cancer. See how easily I can say the C-word now. Am I a better person or not?

My daughter Sarah came in, asked what was wrong. I was weeping. "I want my wife," I cried, "I want Kim." I bawled like a baby.

While her rambunctious third graders demanded attention, Kim gripped her cellphone and calmly said, "We'll get through this, you're going to be okay." She had already been researching other doctors. "We'll find a new one," she said. And from then on, we'd do a better job of directing doctor phone calls to her. She would listen to test results, process the information, determine the next step and most importantly, what to tell me and how. That was our plan.

My harmless bump had turned into a lump that needed to be removed, another biopsy taken, and whoops, suddenly, lurking in my subconscious, with me smacking it down like a whack-a-mole, was a stark possibility that I might lose my ability to talk, to swallow, to breathe... rendered useless, gone before seeing my kids get married and maybe grandchildren, before climbing another mountain, before strolling on a beach in Hawaii, before overseas travel, before Kim and I could enjoy working part-time, traveling, writing and reading, before fly-fishing clear Ozark and Wyoming streams, before haranguing my friends into more crazy adventures.

Chapter Five – Doctor V for Vendetta

A day after the last Doctor Fred phone call, Kim received an incriminating text message sent to her email. It was from her boss, intended for the administrative intern, full of faux outrage, but the intent crystal clear. Put Kim on "another improvement plan" to force her retirement. We had just gone through this nonsense at the end of the last school year, when Kim received her first substandard evaluation in 24 years. We understood, while never publicly stated, that the district encouraged teachers at the top of the pay scale to retire. Encouraged. We would have preferred honest direct requests, help in getting the paperwork in order, offers to substitute after retirement, suggestions for a smooth transition, and a little respect and gratitude for so many years of dedicated service.

Now, however, fully aware of the health crisis we were facing, the boss was ruthlessly going after Kim once again. A colleague was spying on her, reporting every detail that could be misconstrued and reinterpreted.

What prompted this latest attack? Perhaps because we were granted a filing extension for retirement paperwork. Maybe the boss thought Kim might try to stay on longer, perhaps another year, or more. Regardless, we needed the extension to consider looming health costs, the immense difficulty in dealing with family illness, making potentially life and death decisions, and the subsequent need to prioritize and postpone decisions such as beneficiary designation and payment plan options.

Kim finally buckled under the strain and called in sick for the next two days. She went back to work the following week, only to be demeaned and mocked, again.

We contacted Kim's sister Beth and her husband, Brad Ketcher, both lawyers with significant influence, and began drafting a letter to the Assistant Superintendent, asserting workplace harassment and age discrimination. The letter would force the district to investigate and hopefully would force Kim's boss to back off.

Almost everyone has an opinion about teaching because we all have first hand experience as students. Perhaps you are quick to assign blame to teachers. And, after all, nobody is free of fault. Therefore you may think some of this "misunderstanding" must have been Kim's fault. I'll concede that she might have, in some cases, handled the situation differently. For example, she could have worked harder at steeling herself against insidious back-biting and verbal abuse. She could have cultivated the required apathy. But how many great teachers are apathetic?

I have seen my wife teach. I have listened to other teachers praise her. I have seen her students, former first graders, come back years later to thank her. I have listened to her stories, discussed plans and methods with her. My admiration for my teacher-wife increased with each year, as each year she became an even better teacher, an inspirational teacher. (I tried to convey my high regard for her, and for all dedicated teachers, in my fact-based novel *No Teacher Left Standing*.)

I almost welcomed the familiar fight. Her boss clearly led through intimidation and fear, pitting one teacher against another and shifting blame to subordinates. Kim's employment crisis would be consuming under normal circumstances. Between my own teaching and her fight, who had time to consider life-threatening disease?

However, because it needed to be done, I assumed more responsibility for my own fate. I sent an email with a copy of Doctor Fred's reports to our long time friend, climbing pal, MD psychiatrist, and honorary "aunt" to our kids, Lynn Wakefield.

"Today," I said, "I hiked with Sam. Then of course I ran two miles. How can I be sick if I can do all of that? (Please don't answer that. I play games with my own mind.)"

"You're are NOT sick," she responded. "You have some badly behaved cells that need a smack down. Otherwise you are not sick (well, except for that cute little mental thing)."

Maybe I should try describing Lynn in detail. But then she might not want me to reveal all her endearing qualities – her own life has had its fair share of desperately ironic comedy. I met her around March 1978, on a trip to the White Water Races in the Missouri Ozarks. We climbed Mount Rainer in 1981 with John Zavgren. In 1983, John, Lynn, Kim and I climbed peaks in Wyoming's Wind River Range, hiking eight days across the continental divide, running out of food and fuel and near the end of the hike, eating cold, blue grits.

Lynn forwarded my information to our mutual friend, Lisa Caplan, the hard-working president of her company Touchwood Creative providing corporate planning and interactive multimedia. I met Lisa on a float trip, in 1978, when about twenty college-educated young professionals paddled crazily down a high and fast Eleven Point River in the Missouri Ozark National Scenic Riverways, a trip in which I ran freely, nakedly, as happily as I can ever remember running through a field, along the clear Ozark river. Lisa and others watched from the riverbank. After that introduction, I assumed various roles in Lisa's theatre company, The St. Louis Ensemble, and we dated briefly but enthusiastically.

I might sound as if I'm bragging about my friends. But they deserve the praise and I will brag more before this is over. But not that much, because I don't have that many friends. (Who are those people we accumulate on Facebook?) Saying exciting things about your friends is a stealthy way to make your own life sound more interesting, isn't it? And we embrace their weirdness as confirmation that our own insecurities and strange feelings are somehow acceptable; our friends accept that we might have run naked in fields, or paddled vigorously around a bend with boobs gyrating wildly only to have a river patrol emerge from the shrubs with binoculars dangling around his neck and a perverse grin on his face. Some friends, of course, flit on the edge more than others, doing 180s on icy parking lots, hanging out the truck window shooting jackrabbits on the high Wyoming plains with "psycho killer" blaring, eating raw freshly hunted antelope liver while sitting at a crowded bar. My brothers and I have occasionally skirted that edge.

On Thursday January 26, Lisa emailed me. She knew a top-notch surgeon willing to help, who could provide recommendations, and who could follow-up with phone calls. "Please let me know," she wrote, "what you'd like me to do next—I'm standing by."

Between composition classes, I responded, "First, I am overwhelmed with the thought, love and support of family and friends like you. I'm not often at a loss for words, but in this case, I am."

Loss for words? Another cliché. See how bad this was getting?

After a flurry of emails, I had an immediate appointment, Friday, February 3, with Doctor Marc Vavares, director of the cancer center at St. Louis University, residency and fellowship at Harvard medical school, a list of accomplishments several pages long, specializing in head and neck cancer.

Kim was increasingly burdened with excessive, meaningless paperwork, intended to make her employment miserable, so I convinced her that Lynn, who knew the jargon, could go with me to the appointment. It would work out fine. I was feeling good. I'd normalized my life, compartmentalized my emotions. Physically I felt great. I convinced myself that this visit with the super-qualified Doctor V would stop the nightmarish slide into despair and death, and end with a more uplifting diagnosis.

St. Louis University was only a few minutes from the technical college, so no need to rush. Lynn met me in the lobby. We hugged, took the elevator, sat in the waiting room, and joked. Why do these hospitals have so few options for taking the stairs? We went into the examining room where the resident or intern arrived and examined me. Then the main guy showed up with his team, about three white coats.

An immediate contrast to the tentative Doctor Fred,

Doctor V looked me in the eye and introduced himself. I shook his hand, and I said, "I'm gong to beat this."

"That's the right attitude." He asked what I did for a living, was I married. "Who's this you brought with you today?" He shook hands with Lynn, and welcomed her. Then he asked if he could examine me. While his team leaned close, he took a tongue depressor and pushed on the spot on the back of my tongue, and explained to the others that the area was hard. That was the tumor. Then he put a scope up my nose, snaking it into the back of my throat, a step that Doctor Fred had skipped, and one that I would have done to me at least ten more times.

Once Doctor V had sufficiently examined me, he looked me straight in the eye, put a reassuring hand on my arm, and explained his recommendation.

"First," he said, "we need a biopsy, and we can schedule it quickly. If the tumor is squamous, we can treat it with radiation and chemotherapy."

"That doesn't sound fun," I said. "Can't you just cut it out, remove it surgically?"

"We could," he responded, still looking me in the eye. "We would need to break your jaw, then dissect your tongue and split it apart, and then we would—"

"You can stop there," I said, holding my hand up. "I'll take the radiation and chemo." As if I had a choice? Stupidly, I thought he had launched into his grotesque description of surgery merely as a guidance method, and that he obviously wanted me to choose radiation and chemo. So I did. And I blocked all consideration of surgery. Besides, the biopsy would surely show that it wasn't a big deal. I buried the idea that my tumor had already been diagnosed mucoepidermoid carcinoma. Not squamous. Doctor V said that mucoepidermoid carcinoma did not (I think he said "usually") respond to radiation and chemo, so I embraced the idea that it would be squamous. If it were, I would respond well to chemo-radiation treatment. Everything would be okay. No surgery for me.

"It is curable," I asked, "right?"

"Yes."

"Good, that's what I'm hanging my hat on."

Holy crap, I thought, I was using clichés at an alarming rate. In my gut, I knew I was in trouble, but was still having difficulty wrapping my mind around it. Doctor V shook my hand and left with his team. The "patient coordinator" looked me in the eye and very nicely said, "Now there's nothing you can do about any of this right now. You don't need to change anything. Go home and live your life normally."

Outside, in the mild winter glow of the hospital lights, Lynn forced a laugh and said, "Okay, now go live normally."

I should have let out a hearty guffaw. But I didn't. Damn. This time, I was the one missing out on the humor. I merely stood there staring at her, then felt like crying, but was puzzled. Why would I cry? No big deal. A little radiation and chemotherapy and I'd be fine. I had stopped Doctor V from cutting off my tongue, hadn't I? I thanked Lynn for going with me, and we hugged and parted. I drove home, "living normally."

Later, while talking to Kim, Lynn heaped praise upon me for handling the situation so well. I'm not sure I deserved it. Was that me or the Xanax?

The biopsy was scheduled for noon the following Tuesday. After the usual preparations of no eating or drinking past midnight, my daughter Sarah took me to St. Louis University Hospital, and we checked in. I took off my shirt and pants, and put on my hospital gown, then came the IVs. They had me wipe down my body with an antibiotic cloth, explaining that they found it reduced infection rates. I answered the usual questions about my name, age, and what procedure I was getting.

I tried an old joke I'd learned from my WWII hero Dad.

"I'm getting an Opti-rectum-y," I said.

They stared.

"You know. That's when they cut the nerve from your eyeball to your asshole to get rid of your shitty outlook on life."

The joke felt stale while I was telling it. No one even cracked a smile. I told them I was in for a biopsy, and told them I was grateful that they asked such questions. "I don't want you sawing off my arm... or removing a lung."

Still nothing. Not even a condescending smile. Obviously they'd heard these sort of jokes before. Gallows humor elicits honesty. Maybe the most honest jokes of all. Likely, though, they had heard way too much gallows humor from doomed patients.

Sarah sat by my side in the pre-op waiting area. Every time the curtain opened, we could see into an area that looked like a space-age lab for creating robots or half-man, half-Cyborg. What was I to become?

A resident came in and explained that there was a delay, that they might not be able to get to the biopsy until 3 PM. Sarah kept me good company while we waited. Then another delay. Maybe not until 7 PM. This was a trauma hospital.

"If you hear helicopters, then you know it's probably going to be past 7 PM."

Sarah sent text messages to Kim who wanted us to come home. But I wanted to get it over with.

"Don't worry," the resident said, "I've seen Doctor Varvares operate at three in the morning, no problem, as steady as if it were in the middle of the day. He was amazing."

Three in the morning? More than 12 hours wait?

"Dad," Sarah said, "We should go."

Reluctantly, I agreed. Sarah got someone, and the resident returned. "It might only be an hour or so."

But we had made our decision. It was 4 PM. We had been there since noon. We needed to go. I texted family and friends: "Sarah was with me the entire wait at SLU, and I'm so proud of her, the way she handled the situation."

I emailed Lisa and Lynn, thanking them for the prompt action. "While Varvares is clearly the best doctor, SLU hospital might not be the best location for putting together a treatment team given their primary trauma function.... Kim and I are exceptionally grateful for your efforts as we explore every option available."

Kim and Sarah worked hard setting up another appointment, this time at the West County Barnes Siteman

Cancer center. I referred to it as the West County "Difficulty" Center, still searching for humor and my trouble with the "C" word reemerging. The Siteman appointment was two weeks out but the person at Siteman was reassuring, explaining that the wait wasn't going to make a difference, that I had this cancer for a long time. No need to panic. The people at Siteman knew how to handle these situations. So we had a two-week reprieve of sorts in which I could "forget" that I had the big C.

Chapter Six – A Normal Life

I tried to live a "normal" life. But Doctor V's vivid surgery description, halted by my unwillingness to listen, must have been lurking in my subconscious. Not thinking about something obviously doesn't make it go away. While driving back from a run at Castlewood State Park, I had a panic induced epiphany. I shook my fist. I screamed, "Fuck you! I'm not going to die! Fuck you!" I screamed in the cockpit of my car, waving my hands, shaking my fists at the air. A pedestrian stared. Other drivers stared. It was the look people give to the mentally ill. Scraggly bearded homeless people who know the meaning of it all but just can't seem to convey the message to others. Don't you see? You must be mentally ill to see the message. In moments of madness I suppose religious institutions are born, great paintings are created, conquests planned, legends born, and so on. For me, it didn't feel like anything but madness.

I gripped the steering wheel and my shouts turned to murmurs. It was an important moment only in retrospect. At the time, I felt out of control and pissed off. Only in writing about something like this do we call it an epiphany, mainly because we writers are such hacks, trying to make sense of the impossible, trying to organize words around pure fear and anger. What else can we do but try? I suppose if I were 98, I could have shrugged my shoulders and said, "What the hell, I'm going die soon anyway." But at 58, I most certainly did not want to die. Nothing too unusual about that. I had things to do. We all want our lives to be at least partially remarkable, proof that our existence has merit... at least to one other person, someone who understands us.

There were other moments. I hiked and ran my usual

two miles at Forest 44 Conservation Area, and I knelt before the pasture at the end of the valley. "Please God," I bellowed, then fell silent. What would I ask of an indifferent entity that existed only in our imaginations? Weren't my thoughts and prayers nothing more than a bundle of nerves and chemical reactions, positive and negative electrical charges, from stems to dendrites? "Please God. Please God, I'll never..." I stopped again. Never what? Sin? But I'd lived a moral life without God or church or religiosity. So how could this be a punishment? How could this be anything that I had to negotiate with a God? Were my morals based too much on moral relativity? Sure, I'd done some things that weren't exactly church worthy, but who hasn't? There are religious people who I admire, envy to some extent. After all, believers live more satisfying longer lives, at least according to the latest "scientific" surveys. I'd be better off with faith. But even with my moral relativity, I'd done nothing truly evil, or consciously so, nothing remotely like the evil of many religious leaders. I shrugged. What the hell, I thought, so I eked out a prayer anyway. Please God, let me live; I've done some good things and promise to do more.

I did come dangerously close to asking "why me"? I stood in the kitchen and stared at Kim, and said, "I'm not a bad person." But that sort of discussion faded quickly. Didn't matter much if I were a bad person or not, did it? History is full of examples of "bad" people living comfortable, luxurious lives, and "good" people, torturous ones. Wasn't as if I hadn't grappled with these sort of conundrums most of my life. As recently as 2009, a local university published excerpts from my eight-part poem called "The Orange, The Apple, and The Peach," which partly dealt with this concept, "Heaven and Hell are dust / from where we come / and where we have to go."

But, between doctor visits, most of the time I felt weirdly calm, teaching English Composition, grading papers, writing whatever came to mind, running, hiking, trying to enjoy every moment as we all strive to do. I enjoyed my moments with my colleague and friend, Julie Heller. We both started at the Technical College about eight years ago, gravitating to one another quickly, sharing similar interests and humor. It's easy to brag about Julie, a former Air Force meteorologist who speaks pretty good Chinese, who spent a year teaching in Shanghai with her daughter, who has a great husband. Julie quickly became that friend who made teaching easier, and the only one at work who I could confide in about my "situation." We met for a beer in the Central West End. I was fraying at the edges. "It's a total mind fuck," I said. "I don't want to be that cancer guy. You know, the one everybody talks about. 'Do you know that Jeff has cancer. Cancer! Can you believe it? Poor bastard.'"

"You're not that guy," she said, hand on my arm.

But I felt like Tom and Huck peering at my funeral, listening to the eulogy, "And regrettably, Jeffrey Penn May never did get to be the writer he wanted to be."

I felt like shouting from the balcony, "No. Wait. I still have time."

Shoving aside the little problem about my tumor, I helped Kim with her boss situation, and I worked on our precarious finances. We needed to protect ourselves. The 65,000 home equity loan was holding steady at five percent, but eventually it would go up. It could go up significantly and it could bury us. So on February 14, we started the long, laborious post Great Recession refinance process, ridiculously record low interest rates and equally ridiculous tight credit. We made our initial application, hoping to embed our equity-loan into a low fixed rate.

We had gone on vacations with Kim's sister Anne, and her husband John, our kids and theirs, during the "good times," camping at Colorado's Great Sand Dunes, visiting the Southwest and the Hopi Indian ruins, vacationing on Florida's Saint George Island, fishing and swimming in Lake Michigan and kayaking the Crystal River near Glen Arbor. As the economy soured, our vacations became limited to St. Louis and Denver, and then to nothing. Anne got a job with Bank of America, relocating people who were being foreclosed upon. Ironic, some might say, since they were facing foreclosure as well. John started a roofing company. Money was tight, and payments to us were nonexistent. The strain on Anne and John, their marriage, and their three kids, was becoming clear, and I felt like a jerk begging them for our money back. My emails to them were pleading, edgy and frustrated. "Come on you guys, I know you can put aside your own disagreements and think about the family as a whole. One day we will look back on all of this while drinking martinis and have a few laughs. Maybe a vacation in Michigan or Florida or somewhere else. Love from the Mays."

Meanwhile, the secretary at Kim's school overheard the boss screaming into her phone, "I'll tell her I'm sorry! I'll do anything you tell me to do!" Then the boss hung up and yelled, "That fucking Kim May!"

Maybe Beth and Brad's lawyer letter was having an impact. Others were starting to open up, revealing their own less than pleasant experience with "the boss." Through emails, text messages, pizza and beer meetings, all feeling vaguely like Deep Throat political espionage, we learned that the boss changed time sheets to suit her needs, and implemented a scheme with her "boyfriend" to scam money from the district. She talked on her cell phone incessantly, and sent texts during meetings with teachers. She spent more time soliciting compliments on her attire than establishing a discipline program. Discipline was left to the secretaries. She created a toxic environment, using her position of authority to threaten and pit people against each other, colleagues spying on colleagues. Similar to Kim's experience, the principal-boss screamed at the secretary, "I'm your boss" and threatened to fire her.

While Kim and I knew the boss would back off for awhile, we also knew she would likely seek revenge.

Chapter Seven – Wild Siteman

We visited the West County Barnes Siteman center, February 23, waiting in the lobby along with other "victims." In the chair across from me sat a woman with the prototypical scarf over her bald head. I expected her to be thin and gorgeous, a movie star in an unfortunate drama. But she was badly overweight and flipping through a magazine with a lemon cake on the front. This woman's eyes were telling me to Fuck Off.

I suggested we change seats. Kim wanted to know why, but I just said I liked sitting near the door. Which is true. I always liked sitting by the door, so I could make a quick escape. I could run away from this mess and move to Wyoming and fly-fish every day. Sounded good, except for the incessant wind, and the bitter, bitingly cold winters, which my brother Jim assures me are fun, and summers like 2012's hell on earth unleashed, fire and smoke rolling over the normally pristine Wyoming high plains. And of course my tumor problem.

Each time I'd go to waiting rooms at these hospitals and treatment facilities, I'd be amazed. Not because the people were so nice, helpful, and understanding. Yes, almost all of them were, and that was amazing. Or the sophistication of the equipment and advances in medicine, equally amazing. But what flabbergasted me continually was the overall ungodly poor health of the patients, aside from the cancer of course. Poor saps? Was that me? Obese. Wheelchairs. Limbs akimbo. As if I wasn't concerned enough about my own fragility – look at these people! How did they go on? How did they live such miserable lives? Didn't their muscles ache and skin chaff rubbing against the fat? Didn't their stride make their bones crackle in pain continually? But then, and now, I would meet someone who looked unhealthy yet wore a broad happy grin, brimful of good cheer, comfortable with talking about the 100-plus degree heat as if it were good for a picnic. Who were these people and how could they be so happy? I'd been reading enough about neuroscience to know that the brain was capable of putting "happy" in the phrase "fat, dumb, and happy." But it was... amazing! And intimidating. Who was I to bemoan my fate?

We were called back to the examination room. These examination rooms are testing spaces for all of us, the doctor, the patient, the nurse, the intern, the resident, the patient's wife, my wife, who in this case almost never left my side, and is still loyally there for me. Here's a cancer tip – if you get a life threatening cancer, make sure you have a Kim, or a Kim substitute. Great advice, huh? Hard to retroactively establish a long, trusting, and loving marriage. I'm sure all those cancer books that I don't read say something like, "Make sure you don't do this alone, find a Kim."

We waited, and then met the head go-to nurse, Kevin, friendly, laughter ill-timed but pleasant, often loops his conversation back to the beginning and therefore repeats himself. Then we met Doctor Hiram Gay from Puerto Rico, laid back, informative, caring and steadfast throughout the process. My wife was quick to point out that his name is pronounced "Guy." I thought about saying something like, "It's okay if you're gay," but then thought better of it. I sensed that gay jokes would get me nowhere with Doctor Gay "guy." Those sort of jokes lost their humor a long time ago, or at least post 1990s. Not that there's anything wrong with that. In 2012, awkward gay stories didn't seem as funny as they did in 1982 when my Dad set me up on a "blind date." My date and I spoke on the phone, described what we'd be wearing, my eighties slacks and knit tie, her eighties cowboy boots, plaid dress; she smoked a lot, and her name was Gaye Summers. Running late, I rushed into the bar, saw a young woman in cowboy boots alone smoking, marched up to her, stared her in the eye and said, "Hi. Are you Gaye?"

She blinked, glanced around, and said, "Ah, no, I'm not."

When her boyfriend arrived, a big burly guy, she pointed at me. I waited for an excruciatingly long time, but my Gaye date didn't show up that day.

In 1995, when two macho Metropolitan students were brought down to my office for jumping out of their seats and performing a homo-erotic dance, I stared at them, and said, "Look, I have no problem with you guys wanting to show your affection for each other, but please follow all the rules outlined for our heterosexual couples, you may hold hands, kiss briefly, mouth to mouth, but no tongue...." They practically jumped out of their chairs with their gay denials, and never again disrupted class with their dancing.

Through what I thought was an amazing display of self-restraint, I avoided telling these stories to Doctor Gay. That I have included them here can only be seen as sheer desperation. Then we met the chemotherapy doctor, the attractive, physically fit, Doctor Tonya Wildes. If I had to get chemotherapy, I was happy she'd be my doctor. Couldn't make me say I would look forward to chemo, but almost.

I talked to her about running, and how I planned to run my way right through chemo and radiation.

"Well," she said, "You might. We had one patient who trained for a half-marathon during radiation and chemo."

"Really?" I said. "Hear that Kim?"

But she ignored me and talked to Doctor Wildes. My wife can exchange friendly chat with just about anybody, and since everybody was so nice, and we were dealing with life and death, she was on fast forward, mixing small talk with reality, mixing flattery with research, a brilliant interactive display.

Doctor Wildes took us to see where others were getting their chemotherapy, sitting in a room with sliding glass doors to a beautiful courtyard, and she explained how they go outside sometimes. "If it's not too cold," she said, "or too hot." (We had yet to descend into the summer of 2012, days and days of drought and 100 plus-degree heat.) People hooked up to their chemo IVs lounged back in recliners, including the big woman from the waiting area. They chatted as if they were a church group or book club.

But I was confused about the chemotherapy. Hadn't Doctor V said that chemo would be the treatment only if it was the usual squamous. But so far hadn't most doctors, lab technicians, and strangers in the street concluded that it was a rare salivary gland cancer, mucoepidermoid carcinoma? The confusion lingered in my addled mind. But I preferred my confusion to the possible answers. After all, we still needed a biopsy and the biopsy would show that this all was a complete misunderstanding.

Back in the examination room, nurse Kevin arranged a visit to Doctor Diaz who would then schedule the biopsy. "Hmm, let's see," Kevin said, in the computer glow, "We have something the middle of next month...."

Kim pressed him, suggesting that we had already waited two weeks since the aborted biopsy attempt with Doctor V, and that before that we had abandoned one scheduled with Doctor Fred. "Couldn't we get something sooner?"

Kevin went out of the room and returned with a date for the following Tuesday, February 28, 2012. Things were looking up, I thought. No big deal. Couldn't get any worse. In fact, it could get better. People were attentive, realizing that I no longer wanted to deal with this "situation," that we needed to move on it and "get it done."

Chapter Eight –
The Big Biopsy Restaurant

So on February 28, we met nurse assistant Mandy, an attractive coordinator who promised good cheer and helpfulness, then we met with Doctor Diaz, a young brash, extremely confident short guy who snaked the tube up my nose and into my throat, saying that we couldn't really be sure about what we were dealing with until we had a biopsy. His confidence was contagious and we accepted it. He seemed nonplussed about the tumor. Routine. No big deal. Finally someone who agreed with me, even though he didn't come out and say it. The biopsy would surely reveal that it wasn't nearly as bad as everyone else was suggesting. And I repeated what was becoming a familiar refrain, my tag line with doctors, "I'm going to beat this."

Kim and I arrived at Barnes-Jewish hospital on Kingshiway at 6 AM, Thursday, March 1, checked in smoothly, and went to the preparation room. I told them who I was and what was being done to me, the eternal process of proclaiming myself and my treatment, admitting that I had something wrong with me, that I was damaged. They wheeled me away while I thought it strange that a "simple" biopsy was treated like such a major operation.

When I woke in recovery, Kim was waiting for me, and so was her sister Beth. How nice of Beth to come along. She had been there for the PET scan too. I felt fine. No sore throat, no ill effects. Everything was fine.

That evening, I was moving about the kitchen, looking for something to cook for dinner. I was walking in circles, distracted, when Kim stopped me. "We need to talk," she said.

Okay, I thought, but couldn't think of anything hurtful

or stupid that I'd done to her.

She looked at me, and said, "You know I'll love you no matter what."

"What's wrong? It's bad isn't it?"

"I'll support whatever you decide."

"What? Tell me."

So my wife told me what I never wanted to hear but was now our reality. Doctor Diaz sounded irritated... annoyed when he said, "Mrs. May, I had to do three different biopsies. It took three times before pathology could confirm that your husband has a mucoepidermoid carcinoma. The tumor is huge. I am going to have to break his jaw so I can remove his tongue. Then I will have to take tissue from his leg to reattach the tongue and I will have to find a vein to attach it to because the jugular vein on that side has been removed."

And forget about talking and swallowing, I wouldn't be able to breathe properly and would need a breathing tube, and the surgery would be about 15-hours and the operation "was so horrific that some people chose not to have the surgery."

"He said it just like that?"

"Yes."

"Did he really use the word 'horrific'?"

"Yes."

"Then I choose not to have the surgery. What happens then?"

"You'll die."

At this point, standing in our kitchen, faced with "the horror," I didn't think it too funny. Humor does fail sometimes. I've thought about it a lot since then and can't seem to come up with any humor here. We went to the bedroom. Kim held on while I wept – worse than after a Doctor Fred phone call.

I suppose this was something to cry about, but it's all relative, right? Children are killed, maimed, malnourished.

Sam and Sarah came in and asked if everything was all right. Kim explained that we were fine. "Dad just has to get another surgery, and then everything will be fine."

Sarah feigned calmness. "So we'll get the surgery and move on."

"I know this may sound selfish," Sam said, "But could you just give me $500 and I'll move to Columbia. I can't take this anymore. Things just keep getting worse."

"What?" Sarah said, "You can't leave now! No! Not with Dad being sick. You need to stay and help. I need you to stay!" He and Sarah got into a big argument about their respective goals, responsibilities, and futures, an argument I can't recall but both Kim and I felt needed to happen.

When my tears subsided and the kids settled into a compromise, Kim and I started scraping together hope, Kim vowing to "find an alternative."

Then Kim explained the circumstances in the waiting room. "They gave me a buzzer," she said.

"Buzzer?"

"You know, like the kind you get in a restaurant."

"Really, a restaurant buzzer?"

"Yes, I was waiting with a big group of people, all of them holding their... devices... like they were waiting for a table. When it went off, you were supposed to go to a phone..."

"On the wall?"

"Yes, on the wall by the door, out in the open, where people went in and out. So I went to the phone and Doctor Diaz came on... with no 'Hello, how are you' or anything, he told me that he was going to cut-"

"Stop! I don't want to hear it."

"He told me about the 'horrific' operation, then told me we had time to think about it because he was going on vacation for ten days but Mandy could answer questions in the meantime."

"Then what?"

"When I got off the phone," Kim said, "I went to the bathroom and threw up."

"I'm so sorry honey."

"You didn't choose to have cancer."

"You shouldn't have to go through that."

"I called my Mom and Dad," Kim said. "I was crying.

Some guy in a white button down coat, maybe he worked there. He put his hand on my shoulder and asked if I was okay. That helped. He was so nice. It meant a lot to me."

"So," I said, "That's why Beth was there."

"She came right away."

I held onto my wife, on our bed. While it may seem otherwise, Kim hates conflict. In the past, it hasn't been her nature to be blunt.

"I told nurse Mandy," Kim said, "that her boss was an asshole."

Chapter Nine – Quality of Life

We needed help. Lynn, Claire Wooster and Thomas Nadalin came over for what Lynn called, "A meeting of the mindless."

Around 1980, I met Claire and her husband, Bob, twenty years her senior and a sex therapist for Masters and Johnson. Claire and Bob published *Sexual Style* in 1979. They met at a group therapy session in 1960s England where participants were abruptly asked to take off their clothes. At parties, when invariably conversation drifted to what people did for a living, I always offered that I worked on fighter jets, which was interesting enough, until Bob mentioned what he did. Sex always beat jets. An ordained minister, he conducted our marriage ceremony in 1987, and had been there for us when our baby Ben was born and died November 22, 1989. Bob had always been active and healthy, an inspiration, but fell mysteriously ill about ten years ago, and now resides in a full-care facility.

Thomas, who we occasionally and affectionately called Reverend Death, works in hospice care. He knew both Bob and Claire while they were at the Chicago Seminary in the 70s, reconnected about five years ago and now lives with Claire. Of course, I could go on about Claire, thirty years of shared experiences, but suffice it to say, she remains a great fly fishing partner and life-long friend.

We sat around the kitchen table discussing what to do. Kim expressed her frustration at me wanting to avoid details. "He needs to be more involved."

They were talking about me as if I weren't there. Was I already dead? "I don't understand," I said, "I feel fine. I can run five miles. Hike. Bike. I'm fine."

"So," Thomas said, "You've made your choice. You want to live."

"Yes, but I also choose not to have surgery."

"But," Kim said, "You'll die."

Apparently, the people who choose to forgo the surgery, as I suspected, were much older, late seventies, eighties, nineties. (Looking back, as I revise this, regardless of age, I think I will choose death if the unspeakable happens.)

"Okay," I said, "Then let's get it over with. Let's go tomorrow and cut the thing out."

"Is that what you want?" Thomas boomed. "Because if you sign on the line, they'll cut it out and cut whatever they think needs to come out. They don't care. I've seen it. You better make damn sure you are prepared for the consequences. They'll hack away and you'll never be the same."

"Well," Lynn said, "That pretty much covers it."

"Yes," Kim said, "That's what I mean. You have to be involved. I can't make all the decisions."

"Okay," I conceded. "I get it. But I still don't need to know all the details. I have to walk a fine line."

So we came to a workable understanding, a way forward as I tried to live "normally" but a bit more involved in my... condition. Kim spent hours upon hours staring at the glare of her laptop, searching for what she now termed "quality of life," a phrase to match my "I'm going to beat this." But when I heard her use the phrase on the phone or in-person, I invariably panicked. Her "quality of life" refrain, for me, elicited images of me drooling, on high-powered drugs while sitting in a wheelchair overlooking the Grand Canyon with the brakes unlocked. Relatively speaking, I suppose that could be a high quality life. After all, Bob Myners still occasionally smiled from his wheelchair.

My brothers, John, Jim, and Eric, started exchanging emails with me about our Mom. John and Eric had to call an ambulance because she was acting erratically and wouldn't leave the house for neurological tests. At 91, she was showing signs of dementia or Alzheimer's. When John asked me to meet him at my parents' house, I told him I was in no condition to visit Mom and Dad. I should have gone. Maybe I was being selfish.

My "situation" was, as I emailed my brothers on March 2, "getting more 'interesting'... might have to do a big brutal surgery, radiation, chemo, more surgery... and more crap... a bit tough to handle but I'm going to have a beer and go for a run tomorrow. Those fuckers aren't going to kill me yet, fucking bastards."

John emailed his response. "Wow you can get through it and have the right attitude. Would like to join you for the beer."

Eric responded: "Jeff kick that ass. You will beat it. Especially with that attitude!"

Jim responded: "Did you hear any positive news like you heard previously, like it's treatable and you'll come through it okay? Which I'm convinced you will."

On Sunday March 4, I hiked at LaBarque Creek conservation area, then a little more at Forest 44 conservation area. Then I had two gin and tonics at a bar with Julie, who provided a nice stew of sympathy and humor, allowing me to mix metaphors and feel good about going home and having two beers with Kim while going over our refinance, notes and documentation about her boss, and retirement paperwork.

Then I watched "The Walking Dead" with Sam, trying to be normal. But here's another cancer hint. Don't watch a show where a main character has his chest ripped open by a "walker" and to avoid becoming one of the walking dead, has to be shot in the head, the scene especially effective because of his wide terrified eyes and his nodding, giving the others permission to blow his brains out. If your real life is in any way similar to the "really good show," then avoid the show.

I slept fitfully of course, likely because of the alcohol, then went in to teach with a hangover and fighting panic attacks, concealing the big C from the students, and my supervisor, convincing friends that they needed to keep telling me I was going to be just fine. Even if they had to lie, I needed to hear it. All of my family and friends either believed in me or were great liars.

When Kim suggested we try the Mayo Clinic in Rochester, Minnesota, I said, "Yes!" She could've said we were flying to the Congo for a witch-doctor exorcism and I would have said, "Yes!" She made the appointment, March 12 through 14, and I reserved a hotel through Priceline, and started formulating plans for Minnesota fun.

But she didn't stop there. Relentlessly, she continued her research. She spoke several times with our primary-care doctor. He suggested that cutting-edge procedures were often developed in small to mid-size university towns.

Kim found "the DaVinci surgical system." It was used "to perform TransOral Robotic Surgery (TORS) for selected malignant lesions." It was developed at the University of Pennsylvania and FDA approved in 2009. I am convinced that my tumor started its slow growth long before the procedure was available. Kim sent an email to the University of Pennsylvania, "Would my husband's case be a candidate for TORS?"

Her further research revealed that University of Missouri Doctor Jeff Jorgensen in Columbia, Missouri had performed a significant number of these procedures. Kim called and talked directly to Jorgensen. He convinced her, and by extension me, that he was more familiar with TORS than the Mayo Clinic. We were given an appointment for Thursday. We were impressed with their efficiency while at the same time maintaining a relaxed personal approach.

"Why should we waste a bunch of time going to Minnesota," I said, "when we can just drive to Columbia?"

During this harried, desperate time I called Priceline to cancel our Mayo hotel reservations, got the usual circular voicemail, but eventually, surprisingly, an option to leave a message. So I left a message, a voicemail cancellation. Be careful of Priceline. Despite my complaints and my email to the attorney general and Kim's phone calls, we ended up being stuck with the bill of about 300 dollars.

The day before our Columbia, Missouri appointment, I drove to Barnes Hospital and got an MRI. Always a pleasant experience. Lying on your back. Whirring jet-engine noise as you enter the claustrophobic tube. I waited for copies. They didn't have time to make a CD, but were happy to provide the outdated huge MRI slides.

While I hoped my tumor was shrinking, news about my situation was spreading. Out of town friends contacted me. From Chicago, Lin Shook emailed, "I will envision you as becoming increasingly healthy and happy, with the cancer becoming smaller and smaller until it disappears." Lin owns and operates her dance company Perceptual Motion; it's her life's work, joy, avocation, living on a shoestring but entirely dedicated to her art. She and her husband came to St. Louis at least once a year for float trips, camping, journeys into the Missouri Ozarks that deepened our friendship and our mutual appreciation for nature. Lin is a quintessential artist, combining dedication with an air of the unknowable.

Ken Yorgan in Wisconsin emailed: "Just remember, this is probably less frightening for you than for someone like me who's gotten by on his good looks all his life." Photos of Ken reveal his humor. Ken graduated from Logan Chiropractic College and as a consequence became entwined in our St. Louis lives. Ken pushes the parameters of normal. He and John Zavgren designed an awesome wood-stove sauna which we used for years on an Ozark farm near Steelville, the one-time population center of the US. Ken has a razor wit that he isn't afraid to use as a hammer. He is a mental labyrinth. Ask him a question and he's likely to say something like, "I'll get back to you yesterday." A master at mental misdirection, a natural raconteur, all of which makes him fun, maybe sometimes exhausting for those who don't know him.

"I heard," John Zavgren emailed from New Hampshire, "that you have cancer somewhere in your neck? This can't be true! What have you been told? What kind of treatment are they recommending? Let me know!"

"It is true," I responded, "Wish it weren't. So far, two-inch cut on my neck removed nodes and a jugular vein. PET scan and biopsy revealed primary source on back of tongue and throat. Treatment could be all or any one of the following: chemo, radiation, and more surgery. Despite all this, I am focusing on positive thoughts and the love and support of family and friends. I am not going to die and unfortunately for all of you I will still be able to talk. Period."

"Fuck. What a bummer (you being able to still talk)."

My humor struggle was in "full swing," and I was swinging clichés around indiscriminately. I wanted to laugh in the midst of all this sobriety. On our home voicemail, Doctor Diaz left a message, "Ah," he said, "Just calling to see how you were doing... apparently, I left in a blaze of glory.... and didn't discuss everything... Ah, please give me a call."

Chapter Ten – Columbia

While driving along Interstate highway 70, on clear days, you can see the Calloway Nuclear Power Plant's cooling towers billowing steam in the distance. A few years ago, maybe 2009, on our way back from a forgettable trip to Fulton, Missouri, Kim and I decided to follow winding gravel roads up and down hills and past ominous warnings about nuclear radioactive fallout. The last road emerged right in front of the soaring brownish gray cooling towers. Only a fence, barbed wire on top, kept us from driving our small compact car right into the thing. Nobody was around. Not a soul. Creepy. We stopped, got out and stood watching the steam and water spraying. I said, "We could shoot a RPG right at it with no problem. Makes you feel secure, doesn't it?" On March 9, 2012, however, on our cancer induced vacation to Columbia, Missouri, I barely noticed the cooling towers as we drove down the highway, except to say something intelligent like someday we could all be radiated in a Chernobyl apocalypse.

Columbia, Missouri, that's where Kim graduated from Mizzou and lived in a sorority house, where she spent summers riding her bike around town and working at a clothes consignment shop. Columbia, home of the Missouri Tigers, what my wife and kids called Parkway School District's finishing school because most of their high school classmates became Tigers. The University of Missouri, the first school of Journalism in the world, my grandfather one of the first graduates in 1912, his diploma hanging on my wall for years until I gave it to Carrie May, my niece, who received her Journalism degree in Wyoming and is a newspaper reporter. Columbia, where through the tentacles of Facebook, I learned my brief friend-girlfriend of 42 years ago lived, worked in real estate, and helped promote the Rag Tag Cinema. Columbia, where Steve Weinberg lived and wrote *Taking on the Trust: How Ida Tarbell Brought Down John D. Rockefeller and Standard Oil*, and reviewer of my novel *Where the River Splits*.

Now Columbia would deliver me from my difficulty. As we drove into town, we talked about how nice it might be to live in a university town like Columbia "when this is all over," that well-known phrase now creeping into our conversations.

We found the hospital with no problem, little traffic, no crowds, on a beautiful, cool sunny day, a few trees budding and swaying in the breeze. So nice that I suggested to Kim I would skip the usual Xanax. She convinced me otherwise. Regardless of the scenery, a nice day could turn rough on just a few words.

We easily made it on time to our appointment with Doctor Jorgensen, who seemed awfully young, probably in his thirties. We shook hands, and he was relaxed and pleasant. I avoided the joke about how as I get older there seem to be a lot more young people around. (That I've crammed it in here should come as no surprise.)

Doctor Jorgensen already had the PET scan, and we gave him copies of the MRI, then explained our dilemma. Perhaps because he was in a university town and hospital, Doctor Jorgensen was willing to spend plenty of time with us, about two hours by the time we finished. Kim spoke with him about his new wife, and about Columbia in general. Kim told him about our experience with Doctor Diaz.

"Really," Doctor Jorgensen said, "Jason said that? He must have been on drugs."

At first, I classified his comment in the "weird things doctors say" category. Then I think, despite the Xanax, or maybe because of it, I felt some relief. The comment sounded hopeful. It looked like Diaz could be dead wrong. Jorgensen was joking of course, but all jokes have some truth, right?

Doctor Jorgensen examined me, tube down the nose,

stick on the tongue, mouth inspection, as if purchasing a horse. "Well," he said, "We might be able to do it here." Even before I was examined, confidence in this new TORS procedure seemed so high that they had already scheduled surgery for April 2. Kim's research was paying off. But he hadn't yet looked at the MRI. Kim told him that everything hinged on the MRI.

Eventually, he took the unwieldy slides into the other room, and returned with an almost imperceptible chink in his confidence. "I'll get this on our tumor board meeting for next Tuesday. Then I will call you right away."

"But we're still scheduled here," I said, "for surgery."

"Yes," he said, "I'm pretty sure we might be able to do it here."

"I'm going to beat this," I said.

We were out of the hospital before noon, and started our mini-vacation, getting lunch with beer, knocking around town. Kim showed me an old apartment where she and her roommates used to walk through a bedroom to the kitchen, climb out the window to the backyard for barbeques, and went pool hopping at night.

We visited her old sorority house. The young girls who were lounging on the front steps invited us in and showed us around. We saw old photos of past house managers, Kim's picture there, from the mid-seventies. She looked young, vibrant, and attractive. When Kim and I first met, I scoffed at anything to do with sororities, or fraternities. My brother John had tried to get me to join his fraternity at the University of Missouri-St. Louis, but after a few "beerfests," during which guys passed out while young women sloshed beer on them, I wanted nothing to do with it. I was not a joiner. Sure, I played sports, a sort of George Plimpton type, adequate at many things, but not good at anything. (Except maybe soccer.) Not until I reached fifty did I join organizations like the St. Louis Writers Guild and the Missouri Smallmouth Alliance.

When my wife and I met, we didn't like each other much. She thought I was an arrogant bastard and I thought she was a west county sorority bitch. But somehow it worked out and over the years, I've come to fully, if a bit retroactively, appreciate my wife's experiences. While I had lots of on-the-edge experience, like navigating a John-boat from St. Louis to New Orleans, hers somehow seemed more wholesome, college parties and sororities, a sense of purpose and belonging.

We visited the consignment shop where she had worked. The owner, now an elderly lady, didn't remember her, nor would she, having had hundreds of young girls work for her over the years. We visited the school of journalism and tried to look up information on my Grand-pop, James Garfield May. My Dad, Walter Williams May, was named after Walter Williams, dean of the first Journalism school. Photos of my Dad appeared in at least one biography about Williams. We sat outside and drank beer on a deck in the sun near the Rag Tag Cinema where I went in to see if serendipity would allow me to accidentally run into a woman I hadn't seen or talked to in over forty years. The beer was smooth and Kim and I settled into a good time, almost forgetting why we were there, rolling home around 7 PM.

Perhaps energized by the trip, the next day I ran three miles, had coffee, and sat on our deck in the sun trying to fully forget about what was going on. I graded papers and acted as if I'd be teaching until the end of the semester.

Doctor Jorgensen called as he said he would on Tuesday, March 13; however, he had no conclusive response and asked if we could wait, that they hadn't discussed it enough at the tumor board, and they wanted to gather more information before a final decision. That same day, Doctor Diaz's nurse assistant Mandy emailed me, "Can you please keep me updated as to what your plan is? If you are wanting to proceed with surgery with Doctor Diaz I would like to reserve a date."

"Hi Mandy," I responded, "Kim and I really appreciate your help. We have no plans on proceeding with the kind of surgery Doctor Diaz has proposed. Thanks for your patience, input, and understanding."

Meanwhile, Kim taught her third grade class, struggling to ignore the elementary school turmoil, colleagues wanting to know what was going on, loyalists to the principal still spying, her school dividing like a war-torn Middle-Eastern country. But my wife didn't let up on her research, setting up appointments at MD Anderson, and continuing her email exchange with the office of Doctor Gregory Weinstein, one inventor of the DaVinci TORS procedure.

Doctor Jorgensen was taking too long a time to respond and the longer he took, I thought, the more likely he would bring bad news, the news with each doctor visit spiraling toward a dark abyss, a bottomless pit, another "fuck I'm screwed" moment followed by another.

But I was living sort of an alternate existence, settling into weird calmness again. Running. Working. Everything "normal." Since my tongue had been crooked for years, I was convinced that this thing was slow, that if it took ten years to finally become a problem, then it wasn't going kill me anytime soon. In fact, I thought, maybe I should just skip the surgery and treatment. Maybe I'd die, but don't we all eventually.

I was keeping friends and family updated with emails and text messages and told them I "wasn't the type to post these sort of things on Facebook to my million or so 'friends'."

> March 19: You may be wondering what the hell I am doing about my health situation (or maybe not), especially since it has been more than two months since my initial diagnosis. Delays have been compounded by differing doctor opinions, wait times, and doctor/medical "miscalculation."

> Other than acting uncomfortably normal, and finding out how uncomfortable normal still is, I have gone through moments of (for lack of a better word) despair, and gratitude... especially thankful for friends and family, you guys. For someone who has struggled to avoid clichés... you can imagine the "despair" upon finding out that the only truths are cliches. We've had one delay after another. But

getting it right is most important, especially when the treatment options vary from horrifically extreme to not as extreme, as in okay, we can do this. Also, we've had strange "situations."

Doctor number one (Pugliano at St. Clare) kept changing his diagnosis and did not instill confidence. Doctor two (Varvares at SLU) was excellent, but was constrained by trauma hospital location. Was ready for biopsy at noon but never got it and was told it might be 7 PM or even 3 AM if we heard helicopters.

Two-week wait to meet with doctors three (no-joke Gay) and four (hot Wilde) at West County Siteman. One-week wait for biopsy with doctor number five (Diaz at Barnes). Kim informed by restaurant like buzzer and wall phone about horrific operation that would leave me breathless.

A day after my update, on March 20, Doctor Jorgensen called, and told us that the tumor was too big for them to use the TORS procedure. He also suggested that while at first it was slow growing, it might be faster now.

"What would you do?" Kim asked and Jorgensen was speechless, but then Kim asked, "What if it were your wife, what would you do?"

"I'd go with the radiation and chemotherapy... if I could."

I emailed a new update.

Doctor Jorgensen from Columbia called just now and said that it was too big for the new procedure, and it might be faster growing now, started out slow but... that sort of thing. Nobody knows how it will respond to radiation and chemo, but that's a better option than the massive debilitating surgery. We have an appointment Thursday to set up a treatment schedule. So it might not respond... it might... nobody knows. Not enough data. All I can say is that this really sucks and we never seem to get good news. But at least there is an option. If it were you, I think you would go with the radiation/chemo and hope for the best. This isn't going to be easy. But please bear with me, and help me keep my belief in myself from faltering.

Responses once again proved the cliché about family and friends. The following hearty stew of responses is a partial compilation: "You'll be fine, Jeff:) / I was pretty confident you had the balls to handle this project, but your words are a comforting reinforcement of that belief. / The body has an amazing ability to heal itself. My thoughts are with you as always. / There are trails yet to hike, rivers to canoe and beer to be drunk and I will be ready to join you. / You got this, I'm sure of it. / Peace and meditation and your strength to climb mountains is within you and you can and will beat this because you have never been one to back down or sit it out when faced with a challenge. / It's gonna be okay honey. Please know how much we all love you, so don't let go of your belief in the power of the mind. / You will beat this Jeff. You WILL get through this, you will completely eradicate this disease from every cell."

I have often been amused by a phrase Lynn told me long ago, "Sincerity is the key to life. Once you learn how to fake that, you've got it made." But now pretense had been stripped away, my core laid bare, and I thanked them, as sincere as I have ever felt in my life, thanking them for their love and support. But a natural compulsion when standing naked in front of a group, even family and friends, is to reach for some clothing, so I added my ubiquitous explanation for the schmaltz. "Seems like I'm full of hyperbole and cliché, but on-the-edge truth often comes wrapped in cliché."

Chapter Eleven – Kim's Quest

On March 22, we received a detailed itinerary for MD Anderson in Houston that included an appointment with the surgeon Doctor Michael Kupferman, with a radiologist, a dentist, and additional MRI and PET scans. On the same day, we received an email from the University of Pennsylvania. "Kim, Doctor Weinstein agreed to see your husband."

On Friday, March 23, Doctor D's Mandy emailed again, "I was wondering if you were planning on coming back to talk to Doctor Diaz... could I make an appointment for you?"

I sent medical documents to Houston and Philadelphia. I worked on our refinance, faxing financial documents to Community Federal Savings and Loan. I taught my Technical College students the basics of composition, and graded their agonizingly awkward and inadvertently humorous papers. But that couldn't last much longer. Spring Break was approaching and we would be traveling to Texas and Pennsylvania. I told my supervisor I couldn't teach after the break. My last day, Friday, March 23, Julie and I went out for a drink, enough fun to last me until Kim and I expanded on that fun while touring downtown Philadelphia.

Kim never gave up on her quest for my quality of life. (And of course, by extension hers, as we were inextricably intertwined, one in the same.) She was a virtuoso in dealing with me, the patient, the dumb ass who "didn't want to know too much."

She continued her research, reading enough to know that there were no verifiable clinical studies suggesting chemo and radiation would be effective against mucoepidermoid carcinoma. The data so far showed that it had to be removed surgically, then if necessary, followed up with radiation.

However, Kim did not discuss this with me, and I am grateful for that. I was living in a parallel universe where nothing was really wrong, nothing that a little radiation, maybe some visits to Doctor Wilde, couldn't fix.

At some point, during one of our many discussions, I blurted out. "I'm not going to do the surgery!"

"Okay," Kim said. "I'll respect whatever you decide."

"Well," I responded, so very logically, "Would you let someone cut out your tongue?"

She made another appointment at Barnes West County Siteman Center Radiology.

On March 27, Kim drove me to the appointment. "Bring it on," I said. I looked at her. "Come on, this is a good day, it's the beginning of the end."

She kept quiet. She knew better. I had deluded myself, convinced myself that this was the start of my treatment program, that I had made a decision and opted for radiation and chemo. No surgery. I was fairly good at deluding myself, especially with my fiction, which is, if you think about it, the essence of fiction.

Doctor Gay and his team showed us the MRI of the tumor. I tried not to look at it. They told me what Kim already knew. Clinical studies showed radiation and chemo ineffective. They couldn't even shrink the tumor. Surgery first, they said, then radiation. Probably not chemo. They said I shouldn't wait any longer, that it wasn't getting any smaller and it was already extremely large. They assured me that they'd seen big tumors come out and that everything was okay, that I'd be amazed at what the surgeons could do.

I suddenly felt like we were sitting on a bomb trying to figure out what color wire to snip. Instead of feeling like James Bond, confident with wire clippers and astoundingly lucky, I tried to convince everyone that there was no bomb. I looked at Kim. I felt as if I'd stepped off a cliff, freefalling.

They recommended we go see Doctor Nussenbaum, assuring us that we would like him, that we should at least listen to his opinion, assuring us that Doctor Diaz would not be in the meeting, nor in the office, and that Nussenbaum had a good reputation for dealing with patients. I wondered if they withheld the word "difficult," as in, I was a difficult patient. (I can't help but reference Seinfeld here, the episode where Elaine was labeled a difficult patient; perhaps all social experience is a Seinfled episode.)

So Kim made the appointment with Doctor Nussenbaum. We could fit it in just before our flight. "Won't hurt to hear what he has to say." Kim couldn't go with me, having to defend her third grade class from the toxic school wide environment and prepare them for her absence the following week. Beth agreed to fill in for her sister, reminding me to take my Xanax, being supportive and helpful as she had been from the beginning. Beth had responded within minutes of the Diaz buzzer fiasco, made phone calls, helped in research, provided emotional support for Kim, and more.

On Wednesday, March 28, Beth and I went to the 11th floor of the Siteman Cancer Center at Barnes next to Forest Park. Doctor Nuesenbaum was calm and confident, about the same age it appeared as Doctor Vavares. Like Doctor V, he asked what I did for a living, prompting me to think that medical researchers had done a clinical trial about the psychological effects of cancer, suggesting that success rates improved when you humanized the doctor-patient interaction. He placed a reassuring hand on my arm. He examined me, then explained the tumor, offering hope when he said, "I'd be surprised if it were into the jawbone. There's nothing that I can see to indicate that it is."

Likely, I had selectively blocked information about the tumor having migrated to the bone, because at that moment, I felt as if I was hearing it for the first time. So, while his positive words encouraged Beth, I only heard more bad news, another level of severity. It was so close to the jaw that doctors thought it was in the bone, my mind-bubble space-capsule yawing, stomach lurching.

"So that's good?" I asked. "Right?"

"Yes," he responded, "It changes things. From the MRI, I thought it had clearly attached to the jaw."

"Okay," I said, apparently not very enthusiastically. (Because of the Xanax?)

"What's concerning you?" he asked.

I looked at him. I didn't recall any of the others asking such a direct question. It threw me. He really wanted to know my "concerns?" Concern seemed a massive understatement. I was terrified. Unfortunately, my response, while expressed clearly, was also marred by a few tears.

"I'm worried," I said, "that you'll maim me, cut my tongue out, and I'll be unable to breathe, to swallow, or talk, that I'll be useless and better off dead. That's my concern."

"Well, Doctor Nussenbaum said, as if straining to be neutral, "I won't operate on you until your mind is in the right place."

I offered my defiance. "I'm going to beat this."

But I don't think he bought it. Despite his excellent patient interaction, his good news about the jawbone, and his concern for my feelings, I thought he missed the clinical test trial that must have been done somewhere showing that crying didn't necessarily disqualify you from having the right attitude. Didn't he know that I felt better after crying, more equipped to handle this massive joke?

The next evening, Thursday, March 29, after Kim taught all day, focusing on her little guys while her boss focused on discrediting her, we boarded a crammed, cramped, crowded Southwest Airlines flight to Texas.

Chapter Twelve – The Houston Problem

Mostly we relied on faith that our health insurance would pay, as it should because the premiums were exorbitant even though drawing from a large pool of subscribers, the second-largest school district in the Saint Louis area. We were pleased to discover that treatment at both MD Anderson and University of Pennsylvania was considered in-network. We knew that there was a lifetime cap, around a million dollars, but we also knew that the president had passed the Affordable Health Care Act and that at some point lifetime caps would be lifted. Had that occurred yet?

Would our insurance cover flights to Houston and Philadelphia? Not likely. But regardless of cost, we were going. Our savings might be further depleted, we might have to borrow, we might have to run up credit cards, but what choice did we have? What choice if we had no insurance at all? Would I merely live until I couldn't breathe, the tumor so large that I would topple over in the park gasping for air, the ambulance arriving just in time to shove in a breathing tube, and rush me to the emergency room. Would they then start hacking away? Or would they leave the tube in and send me on my way? What sort of system was that?

Fortunately, we had family. Jim and his wife Kathi offered frequent flyer miles and Kim's Dad was offering to pay for our hotel and flight expenses, without interest or the expectation we would pay him back. (We borrowed from him over the years, at low interest rates, and always paid him back, with interest.)

While working for McDonnell Aircraft, I'd often flown into strange cities at night, rented a car and then navigated my way to a hotel. It was never easy, but at least I was young, much younger than 58 anyway. Now I was happy to have Kim at my side (as if I needed another reason) when we landed in Houston around eleven PM, into the wide flat expanse of city lights and dark corridors, and presumably, into bad neighborhoods with large black oil-filled lakes.

We rented a brand new Ford Focus. I started the car and the back windshield wiper came on. We couldn't figure out how to turn it off. Finally, I got out, went back to the office, and asked for help. The attendant fiddled with the steering column, stared in puzzlement at the wiper blade squeaking and flapping back and forth, fiddled some more, then said, "Oh, here it is." He showed me a complex console maneuver.

"Hope it doesn't rain," I said.

Kim read the Map-Quest directions, and I crept along in speeding traffic, the typical out-of-towner causing delays and near-crashes, a big yellow, jacked up flaming turbo-charged Impala swerving around me and peeling out, leaving the smell of burnt rubber lingering and obscuring the exit sign. "There," Kim said. I turned sharply and we were on another road with fast drivers, speeding to one stoplight after another. By some miraculous combination of Kim's directions and my driving we missed only one turn which was easily remedied, and we ended up at the Holiday Inn only a few blocks from MD Anderson.

We climbed out of the car, grabbed our bags, and headed inside. I tried to lock the car. The key's automatic lock would not work. We couldn't figure out how to lock it manually. No buttons on the doors, nothing on the dashboard, no indication of a locking mechanism. No manual in the glove box, or anywhere, the trunk, under the seats, in secret compartments. Nothing.

We carried our stuff inside. While Kim checked us in, I called the number on our car rental paperwork. The guy who answered didn't know how to lock the car either. "Let me check the manual," he said. I waited, too exhausted to point out the irony. "Oh," he said, "Here it is."

I went back to the car and, while I held my cellphone between my shoulder and ear, he directed me to the dashboard. "It should be right there," he said.

"Where?" I asked.

There was a small button with a symbol resembling a lock near the radio controls. I pressed the button and all four doors locked. Automatically.

"Thanks," I said.

He started through his customer service script. "Is there anything else we can do for you today, Mr. May."

"Well," I said, "Just a thought, but it might be a good idea if you put a manual in these cars."

"It didn't have a manual?"

"No. That's why I called you."

We settled in around 2 AM, and woke early, emerging into the humid daylight of Houston, an easy walk to MD Anderson, a city within a city, gleaming modern buildings, a futuristic metropolis of cancer research and treatment. Our schedule for the day was clear: registration, meeting with surgeon, PET scan, finishing up around 3 PM. We were to enter at entrance number two, at 1515 Holcombe Blvd, and take elevator A to the tenth floor and go to the Head and Neck Center. No problem.

We snaked around hallways, went up and down elevators, marveled at the modernity, cleanliness, state-of-the-art feel to the building. We studied maps handed to us at information centers, noting the interconnecting buildings and city blocks that made up the metropolis, and entered a crossover hallway, from one building to another, a long wide hallway like a superhighway. After walking the equivalent of ten blocks to go two, we arrived for registration around 7:30, filled out our forms, got a card with my patient number and the ubiquitous hospital wrist band, then waited for our appointment with Doctor Michael Kupferman.

Even at MD Anderson, the internationally praised world-renowned cancer center, it still came down to "the doctor visit," the moments when the doctor would pronounce his opinion, his diagnosis, his recommendation. What would this surgeon say? I'd overheard Kim and Beth talk about him, and had glanced at a photo of him on the Internet. Beth felt sure that he was "the one" because he was smart and experienced and "so good-looking." Of course I didn't care if he looked like God or Gollum, as long has he had the power to heal. (On the other hand, all things equal, most of us would choose God, I think.)

His office examining area felt high-tech, although the chair was of typical design, like a dentist chair. An intern or resident or second in command assistant prepared my nose with the usual numbing spray, producing instant post-nasal drip.

Doctor Kupferman arrived. He was perfect. He was youthful, kind, and confident, perfect handshake. Perfect dark hair, white teeth, winning smile, and perfect body proportions, Apollo-like. If the Apollo rockets could send us to the moon, then surely he could probe through my nose, view my tumor and declare his discovery, that he could get it out without having to even say "Houston!"

Doctor Apollo noticed my running shoes. "Looks like you've done a lot of running."

"A few miles," I said.

"I know a great store where you can get some new shoes."

"Great," Kim said, never one to back away from a shopping challenge, "what's it called?"

He told her; she took down the info.

"Okay," he said, "let's take a look." Apollo probed me through the nose just like the others, like aliens, abducting me, taking me to their mysterious spaceship, all too real. "We should be able to get this out using robotics," he said.

"Really?" Kim said, "We've been told it was too big. Have you seen the MRI?"

"Yes," he responded, "but robotics would be our first choice."

"What if," I asked, "you can't get it out?"

"Well," he said confidently, "If we need to, we will switch over to traditional methods." He looked at Kim. "Would you like to see it?"

"Sure," she responded.

He wheeled in a contraption of wires and mechanical arms with a screen on it where he showed us a colorful, nearly three-dimensional, detailed video of the tumor. I turned away. "I don't want to see it."

He repositioned the screen.

"Wow, it is big," Kim said. "You should look at this honey."

"No thanks."

"After I take it out," Doctor Apollo said, smiling, "I can write papers on it and be famous and you'll be in all the medical journals."

"Sounds great," I said while trying to sort the truth from joke. "I'm going to beat this," I said.

It felt like we finished quickly, the exam and prognosis conducted with high-tech confidence and alacrity. We shook hands.

"Just let us know what you decide," he said, "We'd love to do it here."

"If we do... " Kim said.

"Just call and we will put you on the schedule."

Simple enough. We shook hands again, firm yet not too firm, his eyes bright, straight into mine with no discomfort, confidence exuding from everywhere, the walls, the building, the massive MD Anderson complex, even from the poor nearly obese man in the waiting room who was missing his nose.

At Apollo's suggestion, we rescheduled the PET scan for the next morning, allowing me to eat without having to wait several more hours. We found a nice cafe with an open veranda overlooking an interior MD Anderson courtyard.

Early the next morning, we went into the gut of the small cancer-fighting city again. As more experienced navigators of the complex, we went straight to the PET scan lab. I knew the routine, more or less. However, probably because this lab was not a traveling scan like the last one, the technicians followed a different procedure. I had to remove my clothing, wear a gown, and sit waiting for 45 minutes, chilly, with the cold contrast fluids flowing in my veins. No lighted photographs of other planets, which I found strange since this place was loaded with space aliens masquerading as cancer patients, technicians, and surgeons. This was after all, Houston, wasn't it?

The scanner did resemble a capsule, but in the hands of this world-class technician felt more like a torture chamber. He positioned my hands and arms stretched above my head. "I had them by my side last time," I said.

"Yeah," he responded, "there are different ways, but this gives the best pictures."

My arms ached and were numbing when he finally whirred me out of the capsule.

At the records department, we arranged for test results to be sent to Philadelphia, then headed south toward the Houston Space Center. (Or as they call it, Space Center Houston.) No sense in sitting around the hotel room. Waiting for what? Kim and I were determined to find some fun in the madness, to make the most of a father-in-law financed vacation, and the free Space Center tickets provided by our traveling British friend and neighbor Dave Lancaster. Dave has been working in air cargo for most of his life, moving to St. Louis about 20 years ago, ending up as our neighbor, bouncing around jobs after 9/11, and invariably becoming popular because of his British accent. Not having anything at all of course to do with his charm and intelligence. About ten years ago, Dave divorced, and we enjoyed observing his dating since then, and his current girlfriend, Kathleen, was a breast cancer survivor.

The Space Center was about 25 miles on I-45, flat straight highway south, but traffic was heavy and it took us over an hour. We stopped at a grocery store for cheese, apple, crackers and beer. I bought an expensive corked wine size bottle of beer, the kind of beer that brew-masters use to compete with wine snobs.

We meandered around the Space Center exhibits, trying on astronaut helmets, crawling through a section of a Space Shuttle, playing space games, and then wandered into line for the tram tour. Sitting on the hard seats designed to inflame hemorrhoids, we rode the tram through parking lots, grass growing through the cracks, small square office buildings, a field with a herd of Texas longhorn. Hard to believe that this was Houston. Command center. World leader in space flight. It appeared run-down, overgrown, off the beaten path, on the flats of southeast Texas. We passed a nondescript building where famous words were heard from outer space. At the next building we got out and walked along the balcony area, able to look down on current projects. It reminded me of the factory floors of McDonnell Aircraft, only instead of fighter aircraft, there were Mars rovers, shuttles, space stations.

We boarded the tram and rode to a rocket park where we stood in front of the Mercury-Redstone rocket, so small, a tiny one-man capsule about the size of a PET scanner sitting atop a rocket that looked more suited for a fireworks display. A path led us into a huge hangar where an Apollo rocket was laying on its side, mammoth, the length of several football fields, the command module big enough for a small restaurant. (Just like my space restaurants in *Roobala Take Me Home*?)

On the wall, a photographic progression of the Apollo missions. And I was feeling good about Doctor Apollo until I stood in front of the Apollo 13 display – in big black lettering emblazoned across the top, Houston, we have a problem. Suddenly, the walls separating reality from my vacation crumbled. "Doctor Apollo, we have a problem, get the knives." For a "more traditional" approach in the middle of the robotic procedure. Traditional meant, as I recalled, the vomit-inducing Doctor D approach. Traditional meant being maimed forever. As I stood staring at the Apollo 13 display, Kim approached behind me, and gave me a hug, reading the next quote, "Failure is not an option." Then she led me into the gift shop where she bought me a NASA Failure-is-not-an option T-shirt.

In the parking lot, where our rental car was baking in the sun, I decided that we should have a little picnic, right away. I grabbed the big fancy beer from the Styrofoam cooler. Unfortunately, we forgot to get ice. While I gripped the hot bottle, prying off the cork, I was thinking that maybe this wasn't a good idea. I should get out of the car. Then the beer exploded like champagne. Foam flowed like a volcano over the bottle rim onto my arm, onto the car floor and the asphalt.

"Boris!" my wife yelled, using an affectionate nickname, developed early in our relationship. I was bad Boris.

"What? No big deal."

"They'll charge us extra if we can't get the beer smell out."

"They're not going to charge us extra."

We cleaned the mess, and while the smell lingered, it wasn't overpowering. I drank what I could of the remaining beer but it tasted bitter, foamy, hot. So I poured the last bit onto the asphalt. The cheese had become soft, the crackers damp with humidity, and the apple was mushy.

But even with those little Apollo 13 mishaps, we were feeling good about our space excursion because failure was not an option. After sight-seeing downtown Houston, remarking about how crowded, flat, and humid it was, we found a family-owned, authentic Mexican restaurant.

Houston was the sort of place you might visit in your retirement, traveling around the USA just to see places you haven't seen before. Maybe worth going to once. Rolling back to the hotel, I felt just as you would expect anyone to feel on vacation, seeing new sights, busy with exploration and adventure. I was having fun. I optimistically emailed a big-C update: "Our meeting with the surgeon at MDAnderson went well. He made lots of sense. He would start with minimally invasive robotic surgery and progress to 'normal' surgery at a level that is only necessary. Sounds pretty good. Much better than the doctor who said he was going to do horrible things to me."

On Sunday, April 1, oblivious to being fools, we drove to Galveston, found a Starbucks near the water's edge just as a cruise ship was unloading passengers, people rolling their suitcases across the busy street, desperate for coffee. The ship itself looked like a low income 1960s housing project lying on its side like Pruit Igo in St. Louis. I took a picture and sent it to Sarah, with the comment, "A place you'll never find me."

She responded, "Ha. Ha. Not your style huh?"

We meandered up the street to the artsy section of Galveston and immediately into a tourist shop. As Kim sipped her Starbucks and browsed forever, I became bored with the clothes and tourist knick-knacks, and suggested that I go for a walk and we meet up later.

I hiked up and down streets more than once, along the docks, watching the gulls and the shrimp boats, watching a crew haul in shrimp, put them in buckets full of ice and carry them to their trucks.

If we thought about money, it interfered with our carefree vacation, and we worried about the meals and rentals not covered by Kim's Dad, worried about paying the inevitable hidden, not covered, insurance costs, and the lifetime cap.

Understandably, neither Kim nor I could afford an Iphone. We navigated by blundering about and looking at the sun. None of the tourist centers had a usable map, so I went searching for one, and hiked out of the tourist zone along a busy street, cars zipping along, drivers looking as if they had a purpose. I found an old "historic" building information center closed because of budget cuts. On my way back, I stopped in an old ice cream store and the generous owner dug through a pile of pamphlets and found me a map. Galveston now lay in the palm of my hand.

By the time I rejoined my wife, we were hungry, passing the usual joints with cheeseburgers, fries, corn dogs, ice cream, and we stumbled upon a Mediterranean style restaurant, ordered a plate of mostly unidentifiable but healthy food, enjoying every bite.

We continued our exploration, up and down streets, in and out of shops, eventually getting hungry again and deciding to look for shrimp. Surely, given the catch I'd seen earlier, the town brimmed full of fresh shrimp. We tried an over-priced water's edge restaurant full of people who spent money because they wanted others to know they had money. The six shrimp were Jumbo, relatively fresh and delicious, and the "cheap" vodka was indistinguishable from all vodka. Maybe the high-class tonic made it taste the same. Turns out the shrimp were not from the Gulf, but were jetted to

Galveston on expensive cargo planes, perhaps justifying the exorbitant prices. I wanted shrimp that I'd seen hauled from the water earlier in the day. We walked across the railroad tracks and along the dock to some low-class place called the Shrimp Shack. While the beer came in massive mugs and the cost was more than reasonable, the shrimp tasted like old tires, chewy and dirty. These shrimp had been frozen forever and flown in from Alaska.

"Think globally," I said.

"Buy locally," Kim said.

We decided to give up on our quest for shrimp, and armed with my map, climbed into the car and went in search of a beach, passing one public beach sign after another. Finally, I turned, and the narrow road led into a subdivision, the public "access" a narrow trail between houses.

After three erroneous meanderings, starting to feel like real estate agents, we found a large suitable beach where pickup trucks and cars had backed down to water, most blasting out country music, side-by-side Texas folk. We found a slot, backed into it, opened the Ford Focus hatch, joined the beach revelers, and watched the waves roll in.

A compact car like our rental was parked next to us, and in one aluminum, colorfully thatched folding chair, sat an overweight couple, possibly in their 30s, she wearing a string bikini, much of it lost in folds. His belly obscured the top of his trunks. She was sitting in his lap. The chair did not seem up to the task. They kissed, and stared into each other's eyes like teenagers. While Kim and I played in the water, they sat, kissed, stared. In the sand, they had drawn a big heart with their names inside, Bob and Isabelle. Felt like at least an hour before the couple managed to extricate themselves from the folding chair – fabric and aluminum creaking.

I waded into the gulf up to my knees and stood. Bob came up to Kim and asked her if we wanted our picture taken. I waded back and joked with him.

"Hey," I said, smiling, "you hitting on my wife?"

Bob puffed up his chest. "No sir, I'd never step in another man's puddle."

What did that mean? I responded with a lame "just

joking" comment. Evidently, around those parts, stepping in a man's puddle wasn't good, and it must have occurred with regularity. But as far as I could tell, Bob was just a nice guy in love. He took a picture of Kim and me kissing in the surf.

After watching the sun sink toward the gulf horizon, we headed back, wanting to minimize having to drive on the crazy Houston streets in the dark. Aside from the funny cancer thing, we'd had a perfect tourist Sunday in Galveston.

Monday, however, we were back at the MD Anderson Metropolis to meet the world renowned radiologist and then the top-notch head and neck cancer dentist.

The radiologist confirmed that yes, likely I would need radiation after surgery and briefly spoke about side effects that I immediately blocked. Then the dentist examined my teeth and said that they were in pretty good shape, only a minor cavity that would need filling and then she explained the fluoride trays. I would have to use fluoride trays to protect my teeth.

"Okay," I said, "I can do that."

She looked at me and very seriously, with emphasis, said, "You will need to use them twice a day."

"Okay."

"For the rest of your life."

"What?"

Trying to negotiate with expert doctors, in this case an expert cancer dentist doctor at the world-renowned MD Anderson, is next to impossible. But I tried. "Well," I said, "my teeth should be nice and bright and white then." Joking, of course, but expecting it to be true.

"No," she said, "Actually, the fluoride makes them yellow."

"Oh."

"Radiation does funny things to the biology of the mouth."

Ha. Ha. Funny things.

After the dentist, Kim and I discussed the "for the rest of your life" comment, me insisting that it was BS, that there was no way I was going to accept it. Using fluoride trays every friggin' day was not the full recovery I was after. Was

I going to stop on the way up a glacier to slip in my fluoride trays? Yes, I harbored, at 58, glimpses of recreating at least one small mountain climb before I truly became too old. That gave me about 10-15 years, I assumed, and no trays would be packed into the wilderness with me. Kim helped ease my mini-panic by assuring me that there was probably some sort of mouthwash that I could use. I filed the dentist statement away, blocking it. Anyway, what were a few dental problems in the grand scheme, how did they compare to the big issues, like talking, swallowing, breathing. Living.

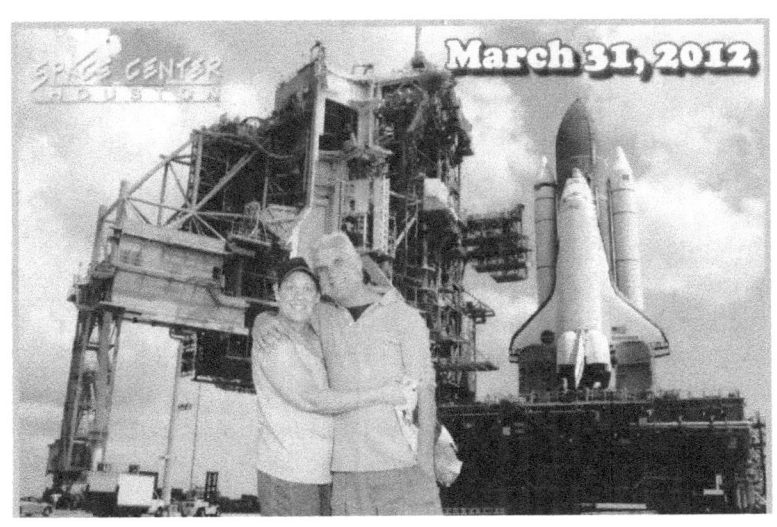

March 31, 2012

Chapter Thirteen – Liberty or Death

On Tuesday, April 3, 2012, we flew to Atlanta, transferred to a smaller plane and flew on to Philadelphia. Kim and I were traveling via air as if we'd been doing it for years. We agreed that having someone else pay for it probably made it easier.

Kim suggested we didn't need to rent a car. We were staying at the Crowne Plaza in the center of town, Starbucks directly across the street, University within walking distance. So we took the train from the airport and emerged downtown, then walked easily through the sunny afternoon, the tall buildings casting shadows and cooling the streets. We would need our jackets here in the pleasant atmosphere of Philadelphia, a contrast to hot humid Houston.

The Crowne Plaza was as you might expect from the name, a relatively classy old downtown hotel, with bell hops, bars, gold colored railings, and red design carpet. Our room was near the top with a window to office buildings. We could see people working at their desks, a world of partitions that I had fled years ago at McDonnell Aircraft. Not that I spent much time at my desk. My boss, a straight shooting colorful German, must have sensed that I was ready to jump out of my skin and quit, go back to one of my numerous strange jobs after college. So he assigned me work that required movement around the factory floor, and from one coast to the other, Patuexent River, Washington DC, San Diego, Fresno, Lemoore, San Francisco, and more.

Now, looking across the great chasm between my hotel and those office buildings, I fleetingly wondered what might have been had I stayed at McDonnell Aircraft, had I not abandoned the "normal" business life and gone into education, leading me to an alternative school full of misfits. Would I have cancer?

I turned away from the ridiculous questions to get ready for an early dinner in Philadelphia as part of our vacation, about as far away from Hawaii as we could imagine. We headed out into the streets, the cool, crisp air, crossing over to the "sunny side of the street." I was tempted to sing, and sing loudly, but usually I only did that when I wanted to punish my children. In my head, however, I was a virtuoso, a pitch perfect Willie Nelson, my voice blending into "Blue Skies" and "Blue Eyes Cryin' in the Rain," a song played by Ron Milburn at his brother's funeral, Thurman dead from testicular cancer. Ron was my john-boat partner on our Mississippi River journey to New Orleans, where my college girl-friend Laury Bourgeois moved and eventually fled to France after Katrina. Thurman was my brother Jim's great friend. I was young. The idea of cancer at that age was inconceivable.

I muttered the lyrics as Kim and I made our way past sidewalk construction, headed North to Rittenhouse Square ringed with restaurants, finding one in the sun and settling in to a great dinner and drinks, again compartmentalizing, this dinner in Philadelphia merely a nice vacation.

Except, for one moment when Kim started talking about how sure she was that Doctor Gregory Weinstein would be able to remove "it" using TORS because he had created the procedure and was the world expert.

Even though Doctor Weinstein's assistant Trisch recommended we take a cab, we walked Market Street, across the Schuylkill River bridge to 34th and Spruce, past university lecture halls, red brick and traditional (reminding us of St. Louis University and Washington University in St. Louis), arriving early at the University of Pennsylvania hospital.

At the crowded sloping sidewalk entrance, in the shadows, a wheelchair bound guy in fatigues smoked, oxygen tank, maimed, as if he had nowhere to go, homeless and just waiting for someone to heal him. I wanted to touch him and avoid him at the same time, wanted to have the power to heal but knew I couldn't even heal myself. And I feared that I might be like him one day.

We snaked our way through the hospital, up an escalator, up to the sixth floor to a crowded waiting room. We checked in with a young guy dressed in a University T-shirt, looking like a typical college Freshman. There were no windows, classic old building with bad lighting, yellowish and dirty, narrow hallways leading to the examining rooms, out-of-style tile floors. I felt uneasy. Despite another vow to forgo the Xanax, I succumbed quickly. We filled out paperwork about the TORS procedure, a rating scale about the patient's ability to swallow, breathe, talk, a sudden realization befalling me that people could have only partial success, that they often got stuck in that no-man's land of being okay but not-quite-right, possibly for the rest of their lives. Even with this state-of-the-art phenomenal robotic DaVinci TORS surgery. Our appointment was at 12:30. It was noon. I had to get out. I asked the kid at the desk if we could wait outside. He said, no problem, just be back at 12:30. In addition, Trisch had told Kim that Doctor Weinstein, like our primary care doctor, often took a long time with patients and therefore typically ran late.

So we retreated to the sunlight across the street, the university campus full of hope and life, and I talked on the phone to my psychiatrist friend Lynn with no recollection of our conversation. When I got off I suggested we should return to the waiting room but Kim said we had time, so we lingered, and eventually returned five minutes in advance of 12:30, but the kid said they had called our name. When we didn't respond, they had to take the next patient. That was the policy.

Waiting this time was excruciating. Was the Xanax failing me? Would we have to wait hours in this purgatory? Kim reassured me, and again expressed her confidence in Doctor Weinstein, the inventor of this new miraculous surgical procedure. Then, before I could freak out, we were called into the office. We met Trisch, extremely encouraging, accommodating and proficient. She reviewed our schedule, several tests including biopsy tomorrow, surgery optimistically scheduled for next week. Maybe that was standard procedure for universities. Scheduling everything ahead of time.

While we were waiting, I saw a doctor hurrying by the open door and glacing at me. I knew it was Doctor Weinstein even though he seemed different than his online photos. A few moments later, he returned, accompanied by the usual residents and assistants. We thanked him for agreeing to see us. Kim talked about what led us to him, about what an asshole Doctor D was.

"You should let that go," Doctor Weinstein said, "we heard about how he handled it, but now that won't do you any good, moving forward. Other doctors will just get uneasy about it and then they won't want to help you."

We talked about his weight loss using a diet similar to the *Eat to Live* Doctor Fuhrman diet. "I lost weight obviously," he said, "but have reservations about the claim that it prevents cancer. There's no clinical proof."

Then he pushed his tongue depressor down my throat, sat back, and said, "This won't come out using TORS."

I was puzzled. How could he be so certain? So quickly? Was it experience? Had he started carving on someone then had to back off and say, "Oh shit! This isn't working!"

The office was dead quiet as he went ahead with the nose probe, quickly and efficiently.

"I know," he said, "it's not what you wanted to hear. And I know you came a long way. I agreed to see you based on your scans, but couldn't be sure until I examined you."

Kim wanted further explanation, and she referenced Doctor Weinstein's academic papers, the idea that with robotics you need to be able to form a square around the tumor. Kim had read one highly technical medical article after another, impressing doctors by knowing the names of their academic papers, and deferring to their expertise because she said she couldn't possibly understand all the jargon and the complexities of their research. Maybe his ego was bolstered, engaged by the conversation. My tumor apparently was too irregular, close to the jawbone, on the throat, possibly extending across the midline.

"What about," I asked, "MD Anderson starting out with TORS and switching over."

"Who said they could do that?"

I shrugged but Kim knew Apollo's name. "Doctor Kuperferman," she said.

"I trained him."

"He was fairly confident," Kim said.

"Well, I disagree."

I recalled Apollo's own ego, about getting published when he got it out, and a comment about how he had been successful up to this point. "So," I said, "Are we going ahead with tomorrow's biopsy?"

"No reason to."

"What would happen," I asked, "if we just left it in?"

"All the horrible things we're going to do to you would just happen naturally."

I was cataloguing his "horrible things" comment into my "crazy crap doctors say" file as Kim stared blankly, unusually speechless in a doctor's office.

Doctor Weinstein must have sensed our disappointment. "Have you considered laser?"

"No," Kim said, "No one has suggested that."

"You two seem like nice people," he said, "I know you didn't hear what you wanted to hear, but I know someone in St. Louis who does laser. He might be interested in helping you. We can call him." Trisch was standing near the door, and it was apparent that the next appointment was waiting. She tried the phone call on the spot, but couldn't reach this someone-in-St. Louis. "We'll email him," Doctor Weinstein said, "and ask him to contact you."

"Thank you," Kim said, "I know you have to go, but could I ask you one more question."

"Sure."

"Is there anything else we can do? I mean, have we covered everything?"

Doctor Weinstein hesitated, "No, you've clearly done your research. It comes down to your attitude, support, and the skill of the surgeon. I can't tell you what to do, but you would have a support group in St. Louis."

After a short discussion about how laser had a longer learning curve for surgeons than robotic tumor removal, thus not many knew how to do laser, we thanked him again, shook hands, Kim filling in small talk as Trisch led us out.

We emerged into the shadows of the hospital, the unfortunate wheelchair bound man still there, still smoking, still mangled. Then we crossed into the sunlight and headed back to our hotel. Kim was down, having felt so sure that Weinstein would deliver our salvation, the walk back for her excruciating. I felt some relief, assuming that our decision had been made for us and that we would end up back in Houston.

Then we did what came naturally. We went to a great restaurant along the park, sitting outside in the sun, ordering exotic drinks, watched people, and discussed lasers, and light sabers, and spaceships and the glorious weather, the numerous restaurants with sidewalk seating, and how St. Louis could learn from Philadelphia. We expressed our surprise at a city we'd dismissed, a city that we likely would have overlooked or even avoided in our travels, the travels that we were planning for when got older, not anytime in the near future. On this required vacation, the good times were interspersed with moments of terror.

I drank something that had two kinds of clear alcohol and green seaweed like substance. Looked healthy, so I had two. Or three. Kim had a few vodka-tonics. We started walking back toward the hotel but then decided we weren't finished with our night on the town. We were staying another day, according to plan, even though all the tests and procedures had been cancelled because there was no reason. We were reluctant to say there was no hope. Maybe just no hope for the TORS procedure. No way the inventor of a procedure who helped otherwise unfortunate cancer victims lead relatively normal lives, no way that he could put a box around my irregularly shaped, rare salivary gland tumor. But that wouldn't stop us from enjoying Philadelphia.

We stopped in an English Pub and sat at a table with open windows, no screens, people strolling by with jackets on, the cool breeze feeling good as we ordered bread pudding, and ale for me while Kim ordered something called a "Gin Fizz." Her drink had a raw egg in it. My ale was thick and served in a giant mug. Our drinks pushed our buzz into an intermediate zone that made us thankful we only had a short walk back to the hotel. I drunk dialed people. I sent text messages. I have evidence for the texting. Julie texted back, "Sounds like you wandering kids are having a blast!" I think Kim was doing the same thing but I couldn't be sure. I took her picture and sent it to someone. We looked at each other and laughed. The bread pudding was superior.

We managed to exit the pub without hurting ourselves and immediately Kim lead me into another shop full of clothes. So I went around the corner to the bookstore and after a while found myself reading passages from John Barth's *The Floating Opera*. A curious happenstance. Nothing mattered, did it? For those of you unfamiliar with Barth, the main character has witnessed the randomness of the universe, most notably in a WWI foxhole, and blows up a "floating opera" because none of it matters. Or at least that was my remembered interpretation. Then I found *Zen and the Art of Motorcycle Maintenance*. It seemed that the only thing I felt capable of reading were books I'd already read in my twenties. As best as I can recall, *Zen* ends badly too. Before I knew it, Kim was looking for me, and I met her on the street to make our way back, feeling hungry again, stopping in at a falafel store, and finally making it back to the hotel where we hurled ourselves into bed in a alcohol induced passion reminiscent of college.

We moved slowly in the morning, and the father-in-law credit card was maxed out, but we were determined to enjoy another day in the city of brotherly love, so we hiked to the historical district, peering through the window at the Liberty Bell, sliding into a tour of the first congress building, then further to the waterfront and the tavern where Franklin, Jefferson, and Adams drank beer, each with their own special recipe. We sat outside in the cool air and warm sunlight and drank the sampler, making our way back, stopping for more food. While strolling along, I was mentally singing, "I've got a tumor on my tongue" to the tune of "singing in the rain" and my brother John called. "Where are you. What are you doing?"

"I'm singing that I have a tumor-on-my-tongue to the tune of singing-in-the-rain and walking around downtown Philadelphia, what about you?"

"That's pretty weird."

"Maybe, but you know we come from the same stock. What's up?"

"Just checking on you. Shouldn't you be having surgery soon?"

"Yeah," I said, "But right now I'm on vacation."

Kim took me to Macy's where we bought a carry-on suitcase because one of our cumbersome duffle bags had torn open, exposing our undergarments. We found delight in buying such a nifty piece of luggage with four sets of double wheels allowing for maximum maneuverability, and I played with it while waiting in a long line because it was super-coupon day at Macy's and piles of women were buying huge pillows and comforters on sale while Kim shopped for a jacket.

I was ready for another evening of downtown fun but Kim flagged. Back at the hotel, while she slept, I emailed my aunt and cousins, finally and officially giving up on Hawaii. "I'm very sad to convey to you guys that Kim and I cannot visit this summer. I have a large rare cancer on the back of my tongue that will require major surgery and radiation. I'm sorry. We were really looking forward to staying with you and enjoying your wonderful state. Love from Missouri, Kim and Jeff." Cousin Sarah graciously emailed back, welcoming us "anytime of year" and emphasizing that this was not a Hawaii cancellation, but a "reschedule. Love and Aloha."

In an email exchange with my brother Jim, we discussed Barth, whom he called "Barf," and *Zen*. I suggested that it wasn't exactly inspiring while all of it good writing and philosophically interesting, "But," I said, "I need someone with a really good laser scalpel."

On Friday, April 6, we took the train back to the airport and flew to New York Kennedy airport for a crowded wait, then onto St. Louis, landing in the evening around 6 PM, our daughter Sarah picking us up, and then finally home from our dotted-with-terror vacation that wasn't Hawaii.

We were home. Kim started researching laser treatments. But she was getting weary. We needed to make a decision. Something needed to be done. We couldn't wait and research and postpone much longer. It had been almost a year since I noticed the bump. And I examined some photos of me cross-country skiing at Forest 44 conservation area, the photos suggesting that the bump started at least six months earlier. Another photo of me years ago with a slightly crooked tongue. How long did I have this tumor?

I've meditated almost daily since college, but now when I meditated, I imagined the colors green and blue enclosing the tumor, squeezing it, and I imagined the tumor shrinking, and I focused on healing. Maybe I could make it shrink with the power of my mind and meditation. Surgery would not be necessary. But at what risk? If my meditation failed, would it be too late, the tumor having grown beyond treatment?

On Saturday, April 7, our first full day back in St. Louis, I received a phone call on my cell. The caller ID indicated MD Anderson. In a moment of courage, rather than handing my phone to Kim, I answered. Apollo himself was on the other end of the line, calling to talk to me personally.

He wanted to help, and he believed he could get it out using the TORS. "We can expand the robotic horizon," he said.

"But if you can't?"

"There is still the possibility we would move to more traditional surgery, but only if it was absolutely necessary."

He couldn't predict if, or when, that might happen. I asked about laser.

"I don't do laser."

What sort of god can't shoot laser beams from his eyes? But he assured me that they could schedule surgery within two weeks, and he still exuded the confidence you would expect from a Greek god.

When I got off the phone, Kim suggested, "I can tell that he impressed you, calling on a Saturday."

Yes, I was impressed. Apollo provided hope. Where no

one else had, at least he provided a shot at having my tumor removed with minimal invasiveness, and MD Anderson was the best cancer center in the world. We had seen patients who had obviously come from all over the globe. Apollo seemed our last best chance at full recovery, of getting the tumor out through the mouth without radical surgery, better than Doctor D's horrible surgery, better than Doctor Weinstein's "horrible things we would do to you anyway," better than nothing. Would we gamble on Apollo? Seemed a relatively clear choice. In retrospect, I wonder if Doctor Kupferman might have been a little overly ambitious, wanting to make a name for himself and write articles. But he seemed sincere, and sincerity was the key to life.

On Monday, we called MD Anderson and gathered more information about surgery dates, recovery times, radiation. All would be best done there, in Houston. We gave them the required information, but held off on making our final decision. "Just call and let us know," Doctor Kupferman's assistant said. One phone call would set everything in motion.

I ordered books about hiking and fly fishing around Houston, and we researched apartments. Maybe we could even cheer the Astros? But that seemed unlikely, especially after the Cardinals 2011 miracle run to win the World Series. Could Houston provide the same sort of miracle? Lance Berkman played for the Astros before becoming a champion with the Cardinals. Maybe there was some Berkman magic left over. And even if the Houston Astros weren't the best, MD Anderson was. So in email exchanges with my brothers Jim and John I said, "Thinking about living in Houston for awhile. Go Astros?"

On Tuesday, our loan processor called with another request for financial background information. I had been filling out forms and faxing them for months. What else could they possibly need? I was doing something positive and productive, planning for a solvent financial future, but I was also ready for this process to end.

"So," I said, "we should be closing soon, right?"

"Well," the processor said, "No, we're a long way from

closing."

"Why's that?"

"We found a lien."

After I expressed my incredulity, the processor explained that the lien was on our title dated from 1996. Of course that was ridiculous because we had refinanced a few times since then and no lien had ever showed up. Kim, having once been a loan processor, was able to identify the mistake, contact all concerned parties and get the loan processing back on track. The title company was so impressed they suggested she apply for a job.

Our family practitioner, Doctor Chao, recommended that Kim take a medical leave of absence. Kim emailed her boss. "My health would be compromised by any return to work in the near future. I am contacting you directly to avoid unnecessary difficulty in finding a suitable substitute. The first priority in my career has always been the well-being of my students. Continuity through the end of the school year is important for their success. I want my students to have the best as they finish third grade."

Wednesday evening, Kim and I joined Julie and Daryl and Dave and Kathleen for drinks and appetizers. As we drank martinis, we joked about lots of things. At one point we discussed diet and effects on health. Daryl was suggesting that diet had little to do with cancer. I leaned across the table, smiled wryly and said, "Maybe, but I think I have final say on this one."

On Thursday, April 12, I sent an update email to friends and family.

> Regarding my current health challenge, first, I apologize. You might think an apology unnecessary, but I can't help but feel a little complicit in allowing myself to get into this unpleasant situation. After all, I have paid lots of attention (perhaps too much) to keeping fit. So at the very least, this is a misstep on my part. Should I have pursued the "signs" (although subtle) with more vigor? But I did ask two dentists. And my tongue has been crooked for years. (Am I a

liar? Or is that only forks?) Someone in passing suggested that a crooked tongue was a sign of ill health, but I felt great, and blew it off as cocktail party chatter.

The support from family and friends has been outstanding. Mostly, I apologize for potential "uncomfortable" moments. But this is an apology based in affirmation of our shared history, long or short, moments in which we have felt kinship and camaraderie, joy in turning our faces to the sun, breathing in the cool air around us, or laughing at the constant barrage of absurdities.

I know you want to help, to differing degrees, depending on your schedule, your own intense lives, depending on what will ease your own distress. I understand that you must protect yourselves first and keep yourselves strong. I want you to be successful and happy. But, in the course of being happy, if you wish to help me, I would of course love it.

Everyone has reacted as well as I could possibly hope for. Everyone has been positive and encouraging. Aside from the skill of the surgeon, this is most important. Send random positive text messages and emails, or check to see if a phone call would be helpful, provide inspiring stories only of people who have made full recoveries. Believe in me. If you're so inclined, pray.

While you are all smart and know this already, and no one has done this, I feel a need to express it here, since we all occasionally fight these thoughts – please avoid the "at least" phrases. At least you'll be able to drool, or you might not be able walk ten paces but at least you'll be able to watch TV, at least you're not dead, and so on. This reductive thinking is not helpful. I need phrases that say, you will return to your previous peculiar brand of normalcy. For example, if a doctor says something like, hey, I think you might be maimed for life, please interpret it as "Jeff, you're in good shape. Your full recovery will take a little longer, but you will recover." There is basis in neuroscience that a full recovery is possible even in some worst cases. Again, you are all intelligent and my stating it here is likely more for my own good. In dire situations, when all seems lost and impossible, it does no good to blurt out or think, we're not going to make it, we're going to freeze to death on the side of this mountain. Better to keep moving. Negative thoughts and expectations merely increase the possibility that the negative will happen.

There's more of course. You could donate your retirement plan or arrive in my recovery room with a brass band, but you'll have to use your own good judgment for that and not my skewed and sometimes sick imagination. On the other hand, I pay for my beer through book royalties... enough for about a six pack a month. Aside from getting a bit of satisfaction every time I see a sale appear on my accounts, anything you could do to boost sales will go into the beer fund for the celebrations after this is all over.

By the time I get through this, I hope to be a better person. If not, I hope to be about the same person as before (unfortunately for you I guess). But in any case, I will make a complete recovery. I may get cranky, I may cuss or flip people off. If you are around, you may not like it. Also, I might get weepy but that does not mean I have given up. Please be patient and I promise I will return to torment you with bad jokes (supplemented with high quality beer) and emerge successfully from this "challenging situation."

I have an extremely large rare tumor on the back of

my tongue, right side, close to jaw. Obviously we want the least invasive surgery. Proximity to jaw makes it again rare and difficult. Re-constructive surgery likely, cut muscles dependent on how invasive, cut muscles make recovery difficult (typing this now makes me tense). After an exhaustive search (mostly by Kim, she's been ultra-fantastic), and trips to Houston and Philadelphia, we have decided to schedule surgery and recovery at MD Anderson in Houston. (Waiting for precise date but have been assured that it will be within two or three weeks.) We will be living in or near Houston for about three months, through surgery and radiation. "At least" I will be able to write during recovery – and it will be a complete recovery.

With all my love, admiration, and appreciation,
Jeff.

Everyone responded positively – the love and support of friends and family. I got numerous emails and text messages.

Jim responded, "With hyper-acute clarity I hear your message... you blame yourself, or say you missteped. That's bull. Everyone would've done or handled it the way you did. Blaming yourself is counterproductive and negative. No apology needed because there is nothing to apologize for. You're going to get through this and yes it probably will be tough at times but you can and will do it."

And from his wife, Kathi, "Using 'we' for you and Kim facing this together was touching and you are one lucky man to have her as your wife."

Beth Ketcher responded, "Your words are a gift to me – honest and so clearly echoing your voice."

From my niece, the journalist, Carrie, "Uncle Jeff, it is my prayer that you will recover, that you will continue to write and inspire and teach — because, after all, writing is what Mays do with emotion, despair, hopes, and dreams, isn't it?"

From Lin Shook in Chicago, "You are such an

extraordinary and wonderful person. Much love to you."

From Dave Lancaster, "Know you are appreciated... you have a strong support team and will triumph.... Let's hike!"

A long email from Kathleen, mentioning her battle with breast cancer, and her Dad who "was diagnosed with a rare cancer that had a 95 % mortality rate" in 1979, and who was "still kicking around in 2012."

Lynn Wakefield suggested that I read *Alive*, *127 Hours*, and *The Life of Pi*. But I'd already read two of the three and somehow reading about cannibalism didn't appeal to me. (Reading and gaining inspiration from nonfiction adventure, endurance, survival stories would come later during radiation.)

From John Reichle, "You have done amazing things in your life, climb mountains, run a school, I fully believe that you will fully recover!" John was an integral part of our 1993 climbing team, leading Metropolitan students six days into the Wind River Range. He and Andi Boyd have successfully devoted their lives to helping others, especially troubled youth. Both worked for St. Louis County Youth Program when I met them in the early 90s and we developed Metropolitan School's outdoor adventure experience, at the time popularly called a "ropes course."

From Andi, "Hiking today and thinking of you. You're strong and yielding in the storm."

Ken Yorgan: "What's the difference between Willi Unsoeld losing a few toes to frostbite and your situation? Well, choice probably plays a part in it, as well as the scenery in the Himalayas having a broader audience appeal than the ICU at some hospital in Houston, but you get my drift."

I responded, "Wish I had a few tongues."

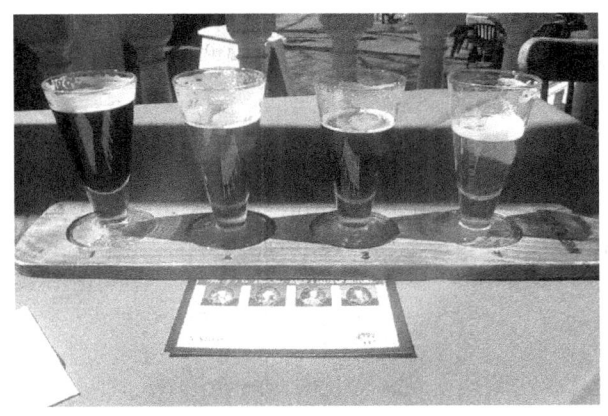

Give Me Liberty

Chapter Fourteen – Miracle On Deck

Of course I was still exercising, hiking and running and bicycling, and eating more or less according to Joel Fuhrman's *Eat-To-Live* guidelines. I went bicycling with Julie and put everything into the effort despite sore hip and back which would fade into sharp insignificance over the next six months, the aches and pains of over-exercising trivial compared to what could happen. Apparently, Julie who is about 15 years younger than me, was impressed. "Amazing job on that monster hill yesterday! I think you might be in the best shape I've seen you ever." And she's no slouch herself, in great shape, running five miles, hiking and biking. And her husband Daryl had laughed heartily at my suggestion that I was the "final authority" regarding diet and cancer. So I'll take credit for that joke. This is a quest, after all.

On April 14, Sarah and I went on a hike at Hawn State Park with my brother John, his son Doug, Dave Lancaster, Kathleen, and Devon the dog, who could barely walk last time Sarah and I tried hiking with him. Since then, however, Devon was diagnosed properly, got medicine, and was acting like a puppy again. I hoped to be just like Devon the dog.

The hike was absolutely fantastic, Hawn State Park on a sunny spring afternoon, water gushing over rock in Pickle Creek, wildflowers everywhere, crisp cool air, wading into fast current and snapping pictures, Devon spraying water on us and stealing one of my socks.

I started receiving emails from cancer survivors, and those who had been "touched" by cancer, specifically head and neck, who apparently, like cancer survivors everywhere, wanted to help. People who knew me only tangentially through family members, who I never met in person. Perhaps this is a bond similar to what I've experienced coming off high peaks, talking with those on their way up or returning, exchanging kind, knowing looks and well wishes. Somehow, however, I enjoyed the climbing more than this cancer thing.

But these new well-wishers didn't know my delusions, my desire not to know too much, to know only what I needed to know. Their emails were sprinkled with words and phrases like "horrible disease" and "recurrence." I skimmed them quickly and sometimes couldn't bring myself to reply, and I now apologize for that oversight, wishing them all many thanks for their concern.

On Monday morning, April 16, at 10:13 AM, Christian Bone, from Wyoming, a friend of my nephew Dan, emailed, and I was immediately discouraged by his first line identifying himself as a "two-time cancer survivor." Two times? Shit. You mean I could go through this again. There was a 30-year span between his testicular cancer and his throat cancer. Shit! You mean I would have to worry about this "for the rest of my life." Over the course of the next few months, Christian emailed gracious prayers and thoughts. One line stood out as a guiding light. "I'll never forget them but the sharp edges of those memories get smoother all the time."

At 10:30 AM, I emailed Anne and John in Denver about the usual financial stuff, "we will be crashing into financial wall around August. We will have to spend rent on Houston apartment, have an income that will be suddenly cut in half." In dark moments, I only knew that $65,000 represented a huge part of my life savings, the little extra equity I'd been paying for twenty years. If I managed to survive, would I struggle financially "for the rest of my life?" John and I discussed his situation in more detail. He had come close to avoiding the collapse of his investments, his accountant eventually saying that he was "toast," and his near suicidal inclinations after that. Everything he had worked hard for over fifteen years came crashing down upon him and his family. Neither one of us were in great shape. I told him that I believed in him, that he would recover from his financial nightmare, and he reciprocated. We will both make a full recovery.

Around 10:40 AM, I joined Kim, sitting on the deck, a beautiful day, cool but not cold sitting in the sun, side by side in our high-class plastic Adirondack chairs. We looked at each other and resigned ourselves to a humid summer in Houston. She gave MD Anderson the go ahead – put us on Doctor Kupferman's schedule. They couldn't provide a specific date but assured us that they would get back to us within the week.

Then came the phone call. 11 AM on Monday, April 16.

Kim's phone played its tune and she answered. I knew enough about doctor phone calls to easily figure out that she was talking to one. More so than any other time, at least as far as I could tell, my panic level skyrocketed. Maybe because the call was unexpected. We had made the decision that we were going to Houston, but this wasn't Houston calling. When I heard Kim use the phrase "quality of life" I fled the house to Forest 44 Conservation area, hiking, running, up the hill, through woods, on my knees again in the valley.

When I got back, Kim was still on the deck, in the sun. She'd had a long conversation with a Doctor "How-ey" or "Hoo-ey" or something like that, spelled Haughey. It would take us awhile to get the pronunciation right, Doctor Haughey, pronounced "Ho-ee." He had a slight accent, from New Zealand, on staff at Barnes in St. Louis. He was at the initial tumor board meeting but admitted that he had been "out of it" from international travel and "wasn't fully there."

"I liked that," Kim said, "He was completely honest. Then he said that he didn't want to upset our plans. He didn't want to make it any more difficult than it already was, but that he'd be happy to see us."

"So," I said, "What should we do?" But knew it was a moot question. I knew we would see this doctor because we never passed up an opportunity for a terrifying doctor visit.

"I think," Kim said, "That we've had nothing but bad news for a long time. And now the universe is dropping something in our laps. We should listen."

I didn't want another doctor appointment. We had already decided our course of action. I was going to be an Astros fan. That was it. It was over. Done.

"I agree," I said, "the universe... we'd be stupid not to follow up."

"Good, I already made an appointment."

"When?"

"Tomorrow at eleven."

Maybe we were turning a corner in our path through the dark forest, emerging from the hedgerows like the ones my father fought through. Maybe we had hacked through a thicket and found a new path, Kim's "quality of life" quest leading us to Columbia, Missouri, to Houston, and to Philadelphia where the doctor saw no point in robotics, but liked us enough to email a world-renowned laser surgeon, and tilt our universe back to St. Louis.

Lisa Caplan emailed me about the "miracle" her brother had hoped for before succumbing at MD Anderson, and I responded, "The miracle in this case may be the strange sequence of events that led us to the only surgeon who might pull this off."

Tuesday, April 17, we met Doctor Bruce Haughey. He was confident, assured, smart, but lacked an overdeveloped ego, no fighter pilot mentality.

"So you run marathons?"

"No. I run, but not marathons. I have done a lot of mountain climbing though... climbed mountains from Alaska to South America...."

"Right then, let's take a look."

He was efficient, working quickly, running the tube up my nose, then the tongue depressor. He leaned away, stared me straight in the eye, and said, "I can get this out through your mouth."

I sat numb, maybe from the Xanax, maybe because I had prepared myself for more spiraling dark, life-ending bad news. What exactly was he saying? I glanced at Kim who was brightening, then having a difficult time containing herself.

"Did you hear what he said?"

"Yes, I think so."

"He can get it out through the mouth."

"Yes," I said, speaking to the doctor, and I suppose trying to be flip, "But can you work with me?" I have no idea what I meant by that.

Since he didn't chuckle, I knew I'd missed my mark, again, cancer comedy elusive as ever. "I'm going to beat this," I said. Although this was the first time it didn't feel like a mediocre punch line.

Doctor Haughey explained that he might have to take some skin and veins from my wrist to patch my tongue. This wasn't news of course. Others had said something similar, only they made the borrowed skin sound more like a substitute tongue. I'd already made a pact with Andi Boyd that if I needed the skin and veins, we would both get wrist tattoos.

"So," I said, "I'll be able to talk?"

"Yes. I should think so. You might have a slight slur," he said, "But you're doing that already."

I hadn't noticed. And nobody else had complained about my slurred speech. So if it wasn't going to be worse than something nobody noticed anyway, great!

"Well then," he said, "we can do it next Thursday. But you can take some time to think about it."

"Not much time," Kim said.

Doctor Haughey and his team exited. We thought about it for about as long as it takes for a bundle of nerves to fire into comprehension, and we scheduled surgery for the following Thursday, at Barnes, in St. Louis.

On the drive home, we assured each other that this was the best option, that this was good. "This is it," Kim said.

"Yes," I said.

Our decision seemed to be affirmed when MD Anderson called and said they could schedule us for May 26, more than a month away. Would we wait another month for an out-of-town chance? Or go next Thursday in St. Louis with a laser surgeon? We cancelled our three-month Houston Astros adventure.

The next day, Wednesday, Doctor Haughey's office

called me, and said they rescheduled the surgery, cleared the operating room for the whole day on Monday.

"Monday?"

"Yes, check in at noon on Sunday."

"Sunday?"

"Yes, surgery will be early Monday morning."

I asked if we could wait until Thursday, so I could wrap my mind around it, but that wasn't going to happen.

I sent an email.

"In a dramatic turn of events, I am going in the hospital Sunday evening for surgery in St. Louis, on Monday April 23."

Dramatic.

On Sunday morning, a cancer survivor and colleague of Kim's emailed, "I have great hope for Jeff. My husband's cousin here in Tokyo was diagnosed stage 4 tongue cancer, operated on in September and is doing well. Part of his tongue was removed and he had to do speech therapy after." She would send supportive emails and cards and would visit, all very much appreciated, but the timing of this information was tough. I didn't need to read I might need speech therapy after my tongue was removed. Wrong image for that morning.

We packed a few personal items, drove to the hospital, and checked in at noon. But my room wouldn't be ready for "awhile."

"Can we just come back at four?" I asked.

"Four should be okay, but no later."

We went to the restaurant PI in the Central West End, ate humus, salad, beer, enjoying our company as we had in Houston and Philadelphia. PI has a sense of infinity about it, eight kicked over onto its side.

We returned at four and were hurried up to a room, given a bed near the door, separated by the usual curtain from another patient, the lucky one by the window facing gray building walls and trash dumpsters in the alley. We joked our way through the usual parade of medical professionals – the nurses, technicians, anesthesiologists, interns, residents, janitors. Then my roommate paced in from the hall, with his gown loosely tied over red boxer shorts, hospital socks, talking on his cellphone, tripping over Kim's feet, brushing past, into his curtained area, suddenly yelling as if the curtain were soundproof, a cascade of curse words. He complained bitterly to someone, a relative perhaps, that "they" were trying to release him but that he was "still in lots of pain," repeating his complaints in varying pitches and a curious mixture of context, syntax, and bad grammar.

I said, "Nice."

Kim rolled her eyes. "Wonderful."

He got off his cell, and grumbled to himself, then brushed past Kim again, out into the hallway to have a heated discussion with a nurse.

"Maybe," I suggested, "We should ask for a different room?"

The nurse returned to check my hookups, and Kim mentioned that the other prisoner was using quite a bit of profanity.

"I think he might be angry about getting a roommate," the nurse said, then left.

"I'll sleep well," I said.

My loony roommate returned, this time going behind his curtain, then pivoting and apologizing. "Sorry about my language," he said, and launched into his litany of complaints.

The nurse returned with orderlies who unlatched the brakes on my bed, adjusted my hookups, laying my IV bags next to me, and suddenly I was on a ride down the hall, Kim trailing, to a different room where I had my own window view to a dumpster, and my new roommate was blissfully unconscious.

After the flurry of reattaching everything, I said, "This is going to be great."

Kim sat staring at me in the bed. "Yes, you're going to come through this just fine."

I drifted off to sleep and remembered nothing before entering a new and bizarre world.

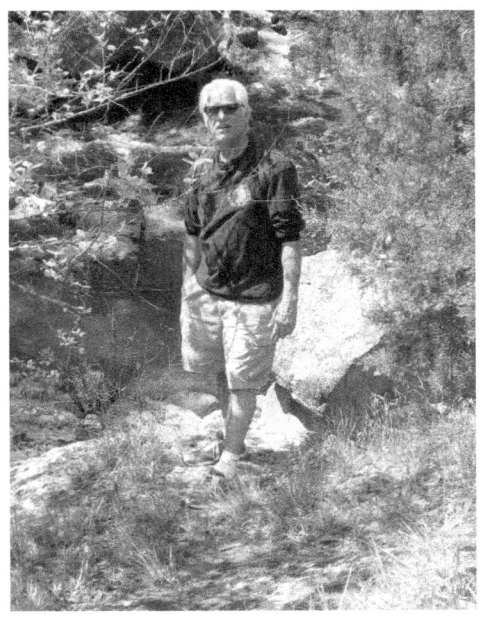

I hoped to be just like Devon the dog.

Chapter Fifteen –
The Big Operation, April in St. Louis

I woke in a dungeon. The walls fluid, pulsating. Dim light, and a weird cacophony, like insects rubbing their limbs together, locusts before a feast. Chains rattled on damp brick walls, and high tech spaceship beeping, or maybe it was a garbage-truck backing into one of the ubiquitous dumpsters in the ally. No windows. Nothing but darkness and shadows. Weird fleeting creatures scurrying from one shadow to the next, making their way toward me. I was alone.

I started screaming.

Suddenly, a lumbering giant appeared looming over me, spikes sprouting from its head, orange, or red, changing in now pulsating light and modulating beeps and buzzes. Words blasted down on me like fists, pummeling me. "You need to be quiet!"

I tried sitting up, and running, running away, escaping, and this spike-headed giant pushed me back down, but not before I saw a name. My face pressed close to a breast and nameplate. April. The cruelest month. With that sudden thought, I held on to a thin thread of sanity. Thank God for T.S. Eliot's *Wasteland*. How could I move on to the more cheery *J. Alfred Prufrock*? Before I could become "a pair of ragged claws scuttling across the ocean floor," my tormentor April, with her spiked orange hair, strapped me down, restraints tight, cutting into my forearms.

"Shut up! You're scaring the others!"

The others? The creeping shadows, the ones scurrying toward me to assist my tormentor? She disappeared and I continued my howling, alone in the torture chamber.

April returned, spring like, a huge lumbering fairy with

powerful hands. "How much do you drink?" she demanded. Drink? Yes, I thought, please give me a drink, anything, something to end this madness. "You lied about your drinking, didn't you?"

Why did this demon want to know? I like most beer – not particularly fond of Budweiser products. Maybe Kim and I drank a little too much in Philadelphia.

"Two," I screamed, "or three!"

"It had to be more than that!"

Was April suggesting I was an alcoholic?

I howled, and I could feel my tongue as if it were unrolling into the dungeon and flapping in the dank air. Would I lose my tongue? I had spoken, hadn't I? Or was that an illusion?

April lifted covers from my legs, grabbed the flesh on my thigh squeezing it in her massive hands, and raised a long hypodermic needle overhand like a knife. For a moment I could see the scene stop in a flash of light from somewhere in the torture chamber. She plunged down, stabbing the needle into my leg, a lovely hallucinogenic experience, like an LSD trip gone horribly wrong.

The shadow creatures suddenly floated into the air above me, while the brute named April with spiked hair tightened my straps, and said something into the darkness, accusing me of having the DTs, of drinking way more than I reported.

To be fair, it's likely I was scaring "the others," although the only others I could see were her floating minions, the scurrying shadows. I was in a real dungeon with April the master torture demon. What was happening to me? If I would have known, I could have calmly said to April, "Excuse me, nurse, my name is Jeffrey Penn May, born 12/27/1953 in here at Barnes for a neck dissection." They repeatedly ask you to tell them who you are and what you're doing there to make sure they don't slit the wrong throat and I appreciated that. "Excuse me," I should have said, "we have something in common. I'm May. And you're April. But I think I'm having a severe reaction to the anesthesia. April, I know we can work this out. Is there any chance we can convene a meeting of my surgical team now, at whatever late hour it is, on April 23, 2012?"

But that would have been impossibly responsible. I'm afraid I acted poorly.

This must be, I thought, how some of my students at Metropolitan school felt when I tried to teach them to at least "act normal." Granted, I did work hard to get their medication right, but they had a lot to deal with. More than I imagined back then. Was it a "failure of imagination?" Would we all be better off if we could imagine the souls of others. I don't know. Maybe. As long as we had control over it. It takes a special kind of person to imagine the plight of others, gain understanding, and effect positive change... without capitulating to the suffering, without having so much empathy that it overwhelms your own soul.

Hmmm. That last bit didn't sound too funny. Maybe I'll need laugh tracks in this. Ha. Ha. You dumb shit, you're suffering from an excess of empathy. Ha. Ha.

April returned again with the needle, this time apparently full of Halodol, a drug my students often took, and again stabbed me in the thigh, and tightened my straps. And for the first time, I believe I quieted. Now I was hyperventilating. I was pulling my arms, struggling to free myself. My left arm had rubber tourniquets with IV needles emerging from my bulging veins.

Kim appeared floating into my consciousness, her hands on my legs. She was kneeling before me, telling me to breathe, "Come on honey. Breathe."

What day was it? Was it the following day? The day after surgery. Was I in a wheelchair? What? I don't know.

Someone who I now call Alverez because I cannot remember his name, changed my tourniquet, chunks of skin tearing off with the rubber. Who was Alverez? Where was April?

The straps had gouged my arm. Or was it the rubber? Alverez said I must have been allergic to the rubber. Wasn't that a convenient excuse? How do I know he wasn't April's accomplice? Hmm?

But it was only my left arm? Wouldn't the restraints

have gouged both arms?

"Breathe," Kim said and I tried pressure breathing as I have done in the mountains, high up on glaciers in Alaska, in Colombia, in Wyoming.

In 1983, John Zavgren, Lynn Wakefield, Kim and I climbed up the snowfield out of Titcomb Basin in Wyoming's Wind River Range. We hadn't seen another soul in four days, nor would we until the eighth day. We crossed the continental divide onto the Dinwoody Glacier, rivulets in the ice melted by the scorching sun, twisting and turning sparkling miracles of ice sculpture, then into the moraine field, forever expanding boulder fields wobbling and tipping as we leapt from one to the other. After a long day hiking over the continental divide, we needed to get out of the moraine and find a camp before sunset.

How I wanted to be back in that precarious moraine field now instead of trapped in my dungeon, Kim begging me to breathe, to calm down, to survive.

I didn't know where I was. What had happened to me? Had I fallen? No, of course not, I was Jeffrey Penn May, at Barnes hospital in St. Louis, for tongue surgery, for a fucking huge tumor. Come on, where was I?

Dave Lancaster and Kathleen Hudson appeared. Strangely, I thought, so soon. Was I sitting up in a bed, or in a wheelchair? Did they bring a card? Balloons? Or just a hello, both touching my shoulder as if I was an old man ready to be wheeled into the furnace and my ashes thrown into the wind, floating across the St. Louis Arboretum Nature Preserve, mingling with the ashes of our first born son, Ben.

"What's with his nose?" Dave said. And later he would say, "I just couldn't get over his nose."

As if that mattered, compared to my tongue, but my nose apparently looked grotesque, the oxygen tube during surgery maybe having torn cartilage, an open wound with oozing blood not particularly fun to look at.

I thanked them for their visit. Had I spoken? It appeared as if I was speaking, which meant that my tongue was still functioning. That would be good. Kim was somewhere with me. I could feel it. Where?

I stared at my forearm. No bandages. So they didn't need a skin-vein patch? Was that good? Yes, I believed so. My tongue wasn't mangled too badly.

But I was in a dungeon. When would I be free?

Chapter Sixteen – The Sixth Floor

The events here are out of sequence, jumbled together, but I am writing them as I think I experienced them, as close to what my memory will allow. Some details I didn't know about at the time, and have been filled in by others, mostly Kim.

That night after surgery apparently I said "Hi" to Kim from my dungeon bed, and I slept all night, or at least remained unconscious. On April 24, I sat up and, according to Kim, said, "Bonanza."

Bonanza? Okay Hoss. Got that. Where was my banana shaped cowboy hat? Are you sure I wasn't asking for a banana. No, Kim insists that I clearly said "Bonanza." Nothing that made any sense, like bandana, or bonsai, or bizarre. Why not something like Steve Jobs "Oh wow!" Or a simple question like, "Am I dead?" How about, "I'm not half the man I used to be." Or what the poet Dylan Thomas reportedly said, "I have just had eighteen whiskeys in a row. I do believe that is a record." April would feel vindicated by that, wouldn't she?

But I make a reference to a 1960s TV show. Adam Cartwright was the dark broody one and Little Joe the peppy youth. Little Joe actor Michael Landon died of cancer, didn't he? So did Steve McQueen. I remember wondering how movie stars could die of cancer. McQueen went to Mexico to take experimental drugs. At his Bonanza hour, his movie star money could only buy a trip to Mexico.

That day, April 24, they took out the breathing tube, and the doctors wanted me to "wake up all the way." I suppose that includes being coherent, perhaps able to identify myself and tell them what they did to me. What did they do? It's possible that my screaming and hallucinations started that night. But I can't be sure. They merely told Kim that I'd had a "bad night."

Time warped. The surgery on Monday, April 23 took 12 or more hours. I remember sitting up with my legs twitching violently, and Kim trying to get me to breathe "normally." And I was moved out of intensive care to my room on April 25. If that's true, then I had three days of dungeon madness that I cannot fully account for.

They wheeled me away. Was it my entire bed or a wheelchair or had I shuffled to my room? Maybe I danced and sang and skipped. Why not? Plausible. What day or hour or decade? (The 1980s decade full of mountain climbing would be good.) I didn't know, but I knew that I had escaped the dungeon, and I had not seen April my tormentor anywhere. Where was April?

Kim would later tell me that she "practically begged" them to move me out of the dungeon.

My room had a narrow vertical window, a sliced view of Forest Park, across Kingshighway, a view that required contortion but a room with a view nonetheless. A tiny room, my bed next to the window, and another bed raised high and crammed so close it would topple over onto me. I saw it wobble and rise and threaten me. I saw its foreboding red light glowing underneath the bed, radiating and pulsating and promising more torture. But none of it was real, just my imagination (running away with me). Imagination, according to my writer-brother Jim, and according to Tim O'Brien in "The Things They Carried" was a killer, especially when crawling into tunnels. Why would anyone crawl into one of those tunnels? Couldn't they just seal them off, bury their enemy mercifully with overpowering blasts which was the hallmark of America at war since the big one where my Dad fought his way through Europe, somehow escaping with his life many times, Bronze Stars, three Purple Hearts, and more. If he hadn't, I wouldn't be here suffering through this ordeal. But we all take our turns don't we? My Dad endured months of death and destruction without a break, often reciting Shakespeare. "Come what, come may, time and the hour runs through the roughest day." My brothers and I avoided

Vietnam because of high draft numbers. Was bad luck catching up to me? Hadn't I paid my dues with Ben's death?

So I kept quiet about the scary bed. And I hoped I would avoid another gregarious cellphone cussing roommate. I had escaped him, and April, and the dungeon. How many escapes would I need to make? Would I get three imaginary Purple Hearts? Now I was boasting again. What I was experiencing had nothing to do with the courage of my father.

My head was bandaged tightly, big wad balled up against my neck, a clear plastic feeding tube curving out my nostril. A band aide on my shredded nose. The doctors apologized about the nose. Since when did doctors apologize? Kim and I were impressed with their honesty, and told them the nose was the least of our worries.

My shoulder and back hurt, probably from my 12-plus hours on the operating table. I was no longer screaming. Had the anesthesia effects diminished? Could I act normal? I was on "voice rest." I wasn't supposed to talk too much so I wrote notes, which made my back hurt even more.

"They think," Kim said, "That you are a flight risk."

I was tethered to my IV pole, like chains, dragging it everywhere. I scribbled on her notepad – Where would I go?

"I don't know, but I think that's why you're next to the nurse's station."

Kim explained my bandages and the voice rest. Apparently, there was a gap in my tongue where the tumor had come out. The wrap around my head, with bunched up gauze under my right jaw, was intended to hold my tongue together so that it could heal that way. No need for a skin-vein patch. But they did use a synthetic mesh of some sort. I wondered if all my screaming had separated the tongue.

Now that I had my own room, I could lie in bed and stare at the vertical slit to the outside. But even under the best of circumstances, I couldn't just lie there. I couldn't stay in bed. I wanted to move, to walk, to scramble over the moraine field, and find camp on the other side of the continental divide. I had to get across, step by slow step. So I wheeled my IV out to the nurse's station, told them, with my

gravelly voice and hand motions, that I was going for a walk.
They nodded, and didn't seem too concerned, probably
because I didn't look as if I would jog out the front door
anytime soon. Flight risk? Ridiculous. As I walked and
wheeled, my arms ached, and my back, especially between
my shoulder blades, tightened and eventually bore into me
with constant increasing pain. I began counting my steps,
something I never did in the mountains. When we climbed
mountains, we endured hardship merely to see how high we
could get, to see how close we could come to the top. Then
we'd return with stories about how "tough" it was. "Brutal,"
we'd say, "but worth it." I tried to imagine each step down
the narrow hallway with the shiny wood floors as a push
toward the summit. Was this worth it?

Kim walked me downstairs for the first time. She asked
the nurse's at the central command center, right across from
my room, if we could go down in the elevator. With
permission, promising not to escape, I wheeled my pole,
Kim at my side, and we crowded into the only available
elevator jammed with visitors, nurses, technicians, doctors,
and the dying. The hospital elevators were being renovated.
So this one was overloaded most of the time.

She lead me down a dimly lit corridor lined with
portraits on both sides, hospital founders, benefactors,
doctors from the past, some staring, one or two smiling, all
aware of their prestige, immortalized and hung here forever.
Without them, where would I be? Houston?

Once through the corridor, I could see bigger windows,
and we rode another elevator down only one floor this time,
to street level, the automatic doors opening magically to the
outside world I'd been deprived of for what felt like eternity,
and I rushed to the railing and sunlight. The air was cool. No
view except to the parking lot, and a few trees and grass, but
I didn't care, and I closed my eyes and felt the cool breeze. I
turned my face to the sun. I'd been in darkness forever and
now suddenly I had hope. If I could return to the trail, hike
high on mountain trails, hike deep into the woods and over
rushing streams, I would live.

There was so much going on inside me that even now I

cannot sort through it. I'm sure that it was hilarious. The best of jokes. Almost cosmic. There was a mysterious noise from the ceiling (or was it the walls?) and it was real. It was an eerie sound as if spirits were whispering (or those shadowy minions?) or electronic transmissions from alien life. They seeped into my room and surrounded me with nonsensical warnings. About what? I listened intently, dismissing my absurd theories. But what was it? My preoccupation with the weird sounds faded because there was something else, something sinister creeping up on me. The lunacy was not over.

Those of you who have spent time in hospitals know that you get no rest. It's no vacation, no long deep sleeps waking to soft rain on trees with clear soothing streams winding around forested bends and limestone bluffs. It's more like constant probing and prodding and nagging, especially with an IV needle. Maybe it's a sleep deprivation test. How does interrupted sleep effect the sanity of the patient. I put a "Please Do Not Disturb" sign on my door, but it didn't work. The sign mysteriously disappeared. Kim thought this was funny, like one of her third graders putting a sign on his desk saying, "Please don't ask questions."

But there was more going on than the usual constant interruptions. I couldn't lie still. I couldn't sit in a chair for more than a few seconds. I didn't sleep more that twenty minutes. I was too hot. I wrapped myself in wet towels in the middle of the night. If I dozed off, nurses woke me up. Time to take your blood pressure. Never mind that my blood pressure was taken a few hours ago and remained as normal as you could get, and I heard more than once, "Wish all our patients had blood pressure like yours."

By April 28, I had endured at least two nights with almost no sleep. My back and shoulder screamed in pain. Morphine did no good. I tried reading but normally I wear contacts and my glasses were designed for distance only. When I took off my glasses, everything turned into a blue-gray blur. Using my laptop made the pain between my shoulder blades worse. Even so, I did manage to respond to a few emails asking how I was doing, one from Robin Theiss, friend and former president of the St. Louis Writers Guild, to which I responded, "Not in very good shape." The other from my cousin Linda who had contacted me a couple years ago via the Internet and who I hadn't seen or talked to in about 30 years. "Been very rough, but okay."

Kim rubbed my feet. She patted my arm. She got me water. She stayed with me into the night. But she was fraying at the edges. I could tell. She told me to "calm down." As if I could. I imagined telling my impaired students to calm down after they'd overdosed on stolen Ritalin. Saying "calm down" did no good. And it was unusual for Kim. She rarely, if ever, said it in 25 years of teaching elementary school. (Exhausted, exasperated, inexperienced teachers might.) Finally, I told her to go away. She needed rest. I was okay. Really. I'd be fine.

Later, I got text message from her. "I love you and tonight I am asking all my angels to please help you get some sleep. I sent you into surgery to get a tumor cut out and I got back someone completely different. Please find your way home. I really miss you."

I promised her that I would stop sending messages, and would sleep, and I wanted her to get some rest as well. But around 1 AM, April 30, I sent text messages. "If I have to endure another night like this, I'll die."

And Lynn responded, "Hang on there, cowboy, Calvary on the way. Claire and I are coming to see you tomorrow."

In the morning, Kim texted, "Did you get any sleep? Lynn and Claire might visit today."

I sent other text messages, although they weren't as imperative as "I'll die." I remember calling my brother Jim, in a whacked out frenzy of back pain, no sleep, feeding tube, IV, voice rest. For no apparent reason, I said, "I love you brother." Other than I suppose, I love my family, my Mom and Dad and my brothers. But it's not something I can recall that we told each other much, if ever. I have three brothers. No sisters. Jim, for his part, was concerned to the point of being physically ill, urging me go fishing with him, recalling all the Missouri Ozark streams we'd waded up and down catching small mouth, sunfish, rock bass, and the Wyoming streams, the huge trout we'd caught just a few years ago when I drove the beat up Grand Caravan 18 hours straight through from St. Louis to Casper. Two days of intense fishing, the trout swirling and turning, attacking, leaping in a horizontal tail flapping visual image burned into memory, as close as I've come to merging trout fishing dreams with reality.

Beth sent a message, "Good morning! Did you move to a new room?" She was going to visit the following day. I mistakenly texted her that I was in room 666, rather than 1606. She joked that she was glad it was a mistake. No doubt there was a room 666 somewhere on this sixth floor. But, if you unleashed your imagination, numerical metaphors could destroy you as easily as reading too much depressing literature. I needed to control my sensitive imagination. No devils for me. Even though I was on the sixth floor and my room number had two sixes, no way I was going to allow a third six. Yes, it had seeped into my subconscious, and into my text message, but that's as far as it would get. Stop, you bastards!

But what was that noise? That almost musical ubiquitous sound sometimes emanating from the ceiling and the walls. Where was it coming from? Voices?

Kim sent another text. "Several people said you texted them last night. I wish you were more sleepy. See you about one. Love you, Kim."

I sent other messages, none of them too cheery, and I was feeling bad about all the worry and anguish I was causing. I leaned on the cranked up tall bed next to mine, thankfully still empty, and painstakingly texted – I'll be okay – wanting to sound enthusiastic. I could get through this okay. I would sleep. Just a few more wet towels at night, and another billion steps, and I would be fine.

On the afternoon of April 30, on one of those rare occasions that I was in my room instead of the hallway, I heard Lynn's voice at my door, followed by Claire's. Lynn had her hip replaced a week before my big operation, and she clanked her walker into the small space. We hugged gingerly and Lynn eased herself into the ridiculously oversized old leather lounge chair awkwardly positioned between the end of my bed and a dresser. Shortly after their arrival, Kim joined them, all of us crammed into my small room.

The room was so crowded I felt more trapped than ever and I kept sitting and standing, picking up books, setting them down, scrolling through my cellphone contacts, and glancing at the door. I paced in the tiny space between my bed and the narrow window. I tried talking, but my words were in staccato, short bursts. For me, my behavior was "normal" because I'd been this way a week, experiencing things in microseconds, flashes of movement and moments. The searing pain in my back and right shoulder continued despite an increase in morphine. (Coincidentally, now as I write this, I have pain in my back, between my shoulder blades, from typing two hours daily as I try to crank out a rough draft before I must return to work in January.) Had I gone from the post-surgery LSD-like hallucinations to frenetic amphetamine-like recovery?

"So, Jeffrey," Lynn said, essential psychiatrist that she is, "What's going on with you?"

I tried to sit on the edge of my bed but bounced off it as if it were spring loaded, and I had no recollection of my ass even touching the sheets. In my darting glances around the room, I could tell that they were all looking at each other, as if something was wrong. Was it me? They were the crazy ones, weren't they? I sat again, and stood up again, and said, "I can't sleep."

"Kim told me that you were taking Ciprofloxacin."

I tried to answer. But Kim rescued me from my incoherence. "His doctors said other antibiotics could cause even more severe side effects, that Cipro was the most commonly used and most effective."

"I'm sure it is," Lynn said, "but for the people who suffer from side-effects, it's not too good. I think he's having a severe reaction to it." She listed several, agitation and sleeplessness as the most common.

Then, as if by grand design, a psychologist rapped on the open door, her name gloriously rhythmic and potentially humorous – Shannon Nana. "Is this a good time to talk or should I come back later?"

Kim took my arm and led me toward the door telling Shannon Nana that it would be great, that I needed to talk to someone.

"Can we go for a walk?" I asked, "That's how I deal with things."

We walked down my billion step hallway and I told Shannon Nana about April and how I felt traumatized. (I remember one of my impaired students using the same phraseology – traumatizing.) We walked, my mind unhinged, unwinding at a moment when surviving seemed difficult. I wept. I was totally fine.

We returned to the room, and Lynn and Shannon Nana had a well-worn discussion about the difference between mindfulness meditation and biological reaction.

"I've called for a psychiatric meeting," Shannon Nana said.

"When?" I asked. Likely there was some desperation in my voice.

"Hopefully within an hour or so." Then she excused herself, leaving me with my guests, Kim and Claire and Lynn discussing my predicament while I wandered in and out of my room.

On one venture into the hall, I noticed a group of doctors with Shannon Nana at a table behind the nurse's station. Things were happening quickly. Suddenly, my crowded room became even more crowded. Lynn vacated the big chair and I sat in it while the psychiatrist Doctor Martin Clarke pulled up a chair across from me. I sat for about a millisecond, then stood, then sat, while he asked questions, methodically going through the possibilities.

I made several lead-balloon jokes about how he looked like a smart guy. Every time he analyzed me, floating treatment possibilities, I said something like, "See, you are smart."

"Do you feel restless?"

"Don't know."

"Anxious?"

"I have to move."

"Why?"

"My shoulder hurts. Takes my mind off the constant unbearable pain."

After several more questions, he concluded that a lot of the manic anxiety and restlessness came from the pain, suggesting Percocet instead of morphine, Seraquil for sleep, Ambien only if necessary. He couldn't change the antibiotic but would suggest the change to Doctor Haughey.

Then it was as if an invisible vacuum sucked all the people out of my room and I was left alone bouncing around and listening to that mysterious sound permeating the ceiling and walls.

Later, Doctor Haughey came by with his team, and sat next to me. "So I understand Doctor Clarke had a visit with you?"

"I need sleep doc."

"Well then, he's the expert on this, we'll go with his suggestion." And that was it. No pretense, no fighter pilot ego. Doctor Haughey reached into his white-coat. "My pen," he said, "seems to have gone walk-a-bout." Someone handed him a pen and he wrote a new prescription, changing the antibiotic to a combination of others including Flyagl, which took much longer to run through the IV, and required me to walk longer and farther, but I didn't mind because I'd exceeded my step count long ago.

That night, I feel asleep. When they woke me up for God-knows-what-reason at three AM, I took an Ambien and fell back asleep. I slept hours straight through for the first time in a week. Later that morning, Julie texted, "Are you getting restless? That's a good sign if you are!"

Chapter Seventeen – Ending April

The doctors roused me every morning, the first one pounding on the door usually around 6 AM, saying loudly "Mr. May, good morning," as he entered asking how I was doing, checking me over, inside my still disgustingly yucky mouth, impressed with the thick disgusting greenish yellow phlegm and thrush. I was constantly bending over my dirty dimly-lit small sink, letting it drool out, forming a vulgar link between my damaged tongue and the drain. I did this regularly, maybe as often as once an hour. I wasn't supposed to spit. Spitting apparently might cause my tongue gap to open up more. I used foam swabs coated in Nystatin to scrub my mouth and tongue.

Sometimes, maybe every three days or so, the early morning doctor took off my bandages. What a feeling of freedom! Air on my head! Occasionally, if time, a nurse gave me a quick hair wash with a shampoo skull cap. Put on the cap, twist and turn. Done.

At some point in this daily routine, the team led by an intent, serious woman who had worked with Doctor Haughey on the surgery, arrived with a team of interns, and peered into my mouth, probing with her tongue depressor. The others looked over her shoulder, sometimes making their own examination, all of them cautiously saying that it was "looking good." I can't remember the names of all the doctors, only that I was always impressed by their professionalism and attention.

Shortly after the group left, if my bandage had been removed, a young, attractive, and short resident came back to rewrap my head, my freedom replaced by more bandages. She wrapped with care and style, a master wrapper, quick, precise, efficient, bunching the gauze up at just he right spot under my right jaw. And, while she worked, she whistled – happily and beautifully. In my ogre voice, I called her "the dwarf." She laughed. Unfortunately, I couldn't talk or communicate skillfully enough to share in the laugh or extend the joke.

When she came in the next time, she didn't whistle, and I apologized for possibly offending her, and tried to elaborate on the Snow White theme. She said that she liked it and had told her fiancé all about it. But this day she was tired from planning her wedding and getting ready for the honeymoon, clearly in love and happy.

My sister-in-law Beth visited often. One morning, anxious to walk, to get outside to the sunny cool air and breeze, my salvation, I waited for her. But she was late. Perhaps, I thought, still confused by the room number. After several text messages, one in which I suggested she meet me downstairs near the entrance, she finally arrived, and we went for our walk. Beth is founder and director of Studio STL, a nonprofit writing center dedicated to helping 6-18 year olds build their writing skills. She had just come from a meeting, with lots of coffee. While I was still on voice rest, she was on high conversational gear, in the meeting problem-solving mode, ending her statements with a question. Not just a yes or no question, but something like, "So do you believe that the European influence on early American writing stunted what would eventually become American realism?"

Kim showed up later and rescued me. They talked and I said nothing, and went for a walk on my own, always checking in at the nurses' station, indicating with my fingers a walking motion, pointing down if I was going outside. I had progressed to walking to the elevator, down the elevator, through the corridor of white-haired patriarchs, and outside with the tube up my nose, and my walking IV pole, all on my own. Such was my independence.

Maybe I could just keep walking around the corner of the hospital to the Central West End, sit at an outside restaurant table, call Kim and ask her to meet me for a late lunch. Dress casual, I would tell her, something similar to my paper-like hospital pants. Bring cash, I would say, because until she got there I'd have to pay them with my pain medication. But how would I get the coffee up my nose?

I pushed my pole, holding onto the monitor that measured the drip of the IV bags. Sometimes, for no apparent reason, the monitor beeped. Not a subtle beep. A loud, alarm-clock beep blaring into the hallways. The random beeps caused me to wheel fast over the hardwood, and steer around a carpet cleaning machine hell bent on its Sisyphean task whirring suds into the dirty carpet. Sometimes, a nurse would appear from a room and press the shutoff button. The obnoxious noise would cease. Mostly, the monitor beeped as it was supposed to, when the medicine finished its drip, and I tried to time my walks so that it finished right next to the nurse central command. Eventually, however, I just shut it down and restarted it on my own. On at least one occasion, I shut off a fellow patient's alarm. Many patients were unable to talk, so they usually thanked me with a nod.

Kim and Beth found my knowledge of monitor shut-off techniques hilarious, and fell into a giggling fit. "Oh nurse May," Beth said, "Emergency on floor six!"

"Yes, nurse Boris," Kim said, "Run!"

They seemed to be having entirely too much fun at the expense of my misery. Then I realized that, while I had missed the initial joke, no way I was going to pass up this opportunity. Cancer comedy was falling into my lap.

"If you two will excuse me," I said, "A patient down the hall needs me to turn off their monitor."

I couldn't tell if they heard me as they were already in a giggle fit, so I exited the room with what I hoped was sufficient melodrama, and off I went on another walk. Unfortunately for me, I missed the full spirit of the "nurse Boris" joke.

During particularly dark times, I remember attempting some humor with the nurses, the usual stuff, asking if they had ever taken blood before, asking where the Jacuzzi was located. I did make one or two jokes about putting vodka in my feeding bag, but stopped because I still could not locate April. She could be lurking nearby with a tape recorder to confirm her suspicions. Or, I could be paranoid. Or a little of both. Who knows?

I got a glimpse of April as I wheeled past a small office at the opposite end of the hall from the elevators, clearly marked on the door, Lead Shift Nurse. The lead nurse was one of three male nurses out of at least twenty. Was there sexism going on here?

I heard April say something like, "I didn't know what to do."

"But you are aware of privacy issues?"

Kim had already told me that the lead nurse had apologized, and assured her that there was nothing in my medical records even suggesting I was an alcoholic. Beth had been there when April was talking to everyone about me as an alcoholic. Beth expressed her outrage in legal terms.

I saw April at the nurse's command center, sitting there chatting with the others, her demeanor relaxed. But I was still convinced she was dangerous.

Another nurse was changing my IV, puncturing a new hole in my ravaged arms, when I asked, "Who is that nurse with the spiked hair?" I wanted to confirm my suspicions.

"That's April."

"She scares me," I said. Then felt the need to explain. "She said mean things to me." It was, I realized, a wholly inadequate explanation, fit for one of Kim's third-graders, but the nice nurse understood.

"They're cutting back staff. She's being let go."

Stunned, I didn't know what to say. Not "serves her right," not "good that dumb bitch," not "hell's minion would go somewhere else to torment the helpless." No, I felt sorry for her. I called Kim.

"Doesn't surprise me," she said.

"I don't want her fired because of me."

"They wouldn't fire an intensive care nurse without lots of complaints. She'll be able to get a job easily. They're in high demand."

So, I thought, I was right, she would torment others. Maybe she would learn her lesson, get a different job, and would understand what to do next time. Yes, that would be it. We all have our troubles. She would get better.

When I went on my next walk, April was nowhere in sight and I was relieved. They'd probably escorted her from the building. My tormentor was gone. I would soon be out of prison, and this whole scary chapter would be over.

Except, near bedtime, she returned to the nurse's station. Judging from her clothing, she hadn't left the building at all. Or maybe she sneaked back in. As I wheeled my IV pole past her, our eyes met. Was that a gleam in her eyes, a hint of recognition? Did she know who I was? Did she blame me for being "let go?"

You hear stories of nurses murdering patients, injecting them with poisons, and making it look accidental. Maybe April would merely smother me with a pillow. She was strong enough. I was weak. I checked my door. Of course the deadbolt lock had been removed. No hospital room door would ever have a lock from the inside. Maybe I could at least push a chair against the door before going to sleep. Then I might hear it scrape across the tile. But more likely it would be one of the omnipresent nice nurses. They wouldn't like it if I blocked the door. But I'd come too far to be murdered now.

I called Kim. "What if she sneaks in and kills me?"

Kim laughed. "That's not going to happen."

"You never know. You hear about it all the time."

"What if there's an earthquake and the ceiling falls on you?"

I took my drugs and slept until I woke at three in the morning of May 1, 2012. I took another pill and made it through the night without being murdered, and that was the last I saw of April.

Chapter Eighteen –
May Is Mental Health Month

My room was no resort. Miniature TVs swiveled from the wall for each bed. At one point, I'm sure these were state of the art, but now were hopelessly outdated. Every time the TV came on, it went to a default video of hospital staff, nurses, technicians, even a few doctors, dancing in a 1980s choreography, stepping like Jane Fonda in her aerobics class, side to side, everyone throwing their hands up in the air like Up With People participants. The 1980s hospital was clean and shiny as if it were new or at least remodeled. The music was intolerable, not even Bee Gee recognizable, something perhaps conjured up by a local synthetic musician group, probably paid for by wealthy donors, all this on a tiny eight-inch screen, the little box on a swivel arm that was apparently supposed to allow the patient to have private access to his or her own little TV. Two TVs per room, with headphones long ago discarded, thrown into the alley dumpsters viewable from the scenic windows. The swivel arms had malfunctioned, like arthritic mechanical arms that refused to move where you wanted, like lifting your elbow to drink and dumping the beer in your lap. Not that I cared about watching TV. Daytime TV smacks of illness. TV means you are sick. Evenings it fills you with too much flashing color and violence to allow restful sleep. (Once I finally got home, however, I watched TV until midnight and took pills to obliterate the overwhelming flashes.) These little matchboxes on the creaking mechanical arms once might have been cutting edge for hospital comfort; however, the dancing 1980s enthusiasm forced upon you by the default channel was now irritating and cutting into my recovery rather than promoting it.

Fortunately, Kim brought my contact lenses and instead of hulking down the hallway with my glasses shoved behind the bandages, ill-fitting and smeared, my contacts allowed relatively clear interaction with my surroundings.

Kim's brother, Dave Einig, visited with his usual fast-paced high intensity, bringing me a book, *Great Plains*, talking fast about what great writing it was and how you could just open it up and read it anywhere and enjoy it. I was pretty sure I'd read it before, but agreed that it was perfect for here. It was great to have Dave's unique energy pumped into my small hospital room surroundings.

While he talked fast, he also listened when I slowly described some of the fun hospital resort activities, my voice rest requirement easing.

"Just remember," he said, "The end is near."

I looked at him. "Maybe you could phrase that differently."

We took a walk, and I lead him around on my usual tour, outside past the wheelchair bound oxygen tank invalids puffing away directly under the big blue and white signs – For the Health of our Patients and Visitors this is a Smoke Free Hospital Campus. Dave wanted to smoke, but I suggested we go further away, and led him to a small courtyard with concealing plants on the far side of the building where he could smoke his "American Spirit – all natural" cigarette.

We returned and watched the Cardinals on the matchbox TV, Dave having no problems seeing it. But my contacts had accumulated gunk and the TV had become, once again, a bit of a blur. I decided to take out my contacts and put my glasses back on.

Standing at the sink near the door and next to the tiny toilet shower area, I looked in the mirror and smiled grimly. I was a sight, scraggly beard growing around the bandages, hair sticking out, and I leaned over the sink that I had been spitting and drooling in. I laid out some paper towels, leaned over and took out my right lens, then I popped out the left one, but it didn't appear in my hand or in the sink. It must have grown moth wings and flown, as contacts sometimes do, landing on the floor somewhere. Usually, I can find them quickly. I went to my knees and looked. The floor was filthy, despite the daily mopping, the old tile impossible to clean.

I couldn't find my contact lens. I told Dave. He came over but couldn't find it. I asked the nurse for help. The only flashlight she could find was suitable for a key chain. "I wouldn't spend too much time down there," she said. Clearly, the filthy floor was a topic, and it was obvious the rooms needed renovation. Finally, given the events of the past months, losing a contact began to pale in comparison, and the search no longer seemed worth it. But I bemoaned going back to the glasses and called Kim asking her to bring an extra lens when she visited the next day.

The Cardinals were pummeling the Pittsburgh Pirates, and Dave mused about hopping on the Metro-Link and going downtown to watch the rest of the game live. I told him it sounded like a grand idea. "However," I said, "You'll have to go by yourself." I did walk out with him, down the elevator, past the ghostly patriarchs, to the escalator, outside, and east, where he immediately lit up another of his all natural cigarettes. They're fine, probably good for him, no way he'll end up with holes in this throat.

This was our second long walk, but I kept pace, walking outside to the courtyard, before we parted ways, and I wished him a good time, then wheeled my IV pole back to the 6th floor. While I wouldn't find out for a few days, it turns out he made it to the game and bought a ticket from a scalper, getting front row behind home plate, and watched the continued pummeling of the Pirates. That's Dave Einig, I thought, living his full life, both highs and lows.

I was tired. After wheeling my pole back to my room, I stood trying to watch the baseball game. I never could get the mechanical arm to adjust for bed viewing, so I stood pressing my face close to the miniscule screen. It was dusk, probably around 8:30. I ached for sleep because I was happy asleep. I turned off the game, curled onto the bed, slipping slowly into semi-consciousness, interrupted by a nurse who wanted to extract more blood from my arms that were busied pincushions.

I turned the TV back on and endured the sudden blasting of that hospital dance routine before finding the baseball game again. Like a failed relief pitcher weary after only one inning, I turned it off. I was finished for the night. No way would I endure the default disco again.

Then I had a theory. Perhaps, I thought, that strange wall and ceiling whispering voice-noise came from other rooms, other patients being tortured with the blaring disco hop beat, the music muffled by the walls just enough to make it seem like a spirit. But straining to confirm my theory, to recognize that obnoxious music, was worse than never knowing where the whisper came from. Aliens. That was a good enough answer.

I went to the dirty sink, moistened a paper towel, and carefully wiped each exposed section of my face. My forehead, over and under my eyes.

I had crawled around the floor, had watched baseball, gone to the hallway and nurses station, walked through the hospital, down six floors, outside, walking with intense Dave, then turned around back to my room, watched more baseball, laid down, tried to sleep, had my blood taken, watched more baseball, and only then, when I washed up, did I see –stuck to my skin under my left eye – my contact lens. What were the chances? Were they one in 20,000, the same as when my son Ben died?

Chapter Nineteen – Protocol

Kim was still working hard at coordinating my visitors. "How much do you pay them?" I asked.

"Not much," she joked, "Usually, they're good with a cup of coffee and a hundred dollars."

During the 12-hour surgery, Sarah and her best friend Dominic, Kim, Beth, and my oldest brother John endured the waiting room, Kim sending text message updates to others. John also visited during my post-surgery hallucinogenic period, although I have no recollection of it. No doubt he was one of the demons. He was also there when I was bouncing out of my bed and wearing wet towels. Or so he says. I'm not giving him full credit for being a good brother until he coughs up at least a six pack of premium beer and agrees to drive every time we go fishing. But I easily remembered him popping in near the end of my Barnes Hospital vacation.

"Nice of you to come by," I said, "Finally."

"Finally? You've been a real pain in ass."

"What? You were here before?"

"Watching you flop around like sucker on a stream bank."

"I'll have to ask Kim for confirmation."

"Now that it's obvious your fine, I'm done with this resort."

"Yeah, I guess I dodged a bullet," I said, "but that seems like a huge understatement." I was apparently so adept at clichés by now that I could use two in one sentence.

Jim of course could only offer long-distance support because he lives in Wyoming, even though he offered to fly in, but there seemed no point in him experiencing my whacked-out surgery induced insanity first hand, which explains why I called him on my cellphone and blathered weird crap to him.

My younger bother Eric, who I had bailed out of jams many times over the years, stopped in. My main concern with him, however, was how he arrived there. He wasn't supposed to drive. Eric's life is a complex story in itself. But it was only a year or so ago that John and I took him to a rehab program where they immediately sent him to this same hospital to have a hole drilled into his head. Of course, we couldn't pass up commenting that he had holes in his head already. My including it here again exemplifies my struggle for comedy. But on a lighter note, it also gives me an opportunity to admit guilt. When I was ten, and Eric two, I set him on our top bunk bed railing, and he flipped backwards onto the concrete floor. All his difficulties could be my fault.

My kids visited. This was the most uplifting of all visits. I didn't realize it would be, but I felt rejuvenated when walking around the hospital, everywhere I could go with them, down corridors, outside, even starting to jog, happily tilting my IV pole forward like a musket, charging my way past hospital guards. Sarah yelled for me to stop, "You're not hurting yourself while I'm in charge." I was sorry to see them leave but immensely grateful. I would not have wanted them to visit more than once however. They needed to live their lives as normally as possible without having this big C thing interfere with their stalled plans any more than it already had.

John Reichle visited early one morning, and I wrote a note to him, telling him that I was going to write a book called *Two Hundred Steps*. Of course now we are well removed from that wholly inadequate title.

Dave Lancaster came by again, relieved that my nose was slightly less grotesque. Using adhesive tape, I had attached a poster to the wall. Kathleen had made it, Sarah providing photos of our Hawn State Park hike not all that long ago. It had bright green lettering – Let's get back to it. Apparently, Dave and Kathleen had given me the poster when I was in Bonanza-land. But, in my retroactive memory, it appeared only just now with Dave's second visit.

Julie texted, asking if it was okay to stop by, but I told her not to, which in retrospect was probably a mistake, as she would have lifted my spirits with her warmth and humor. Perhaps because we were colleagues, I didn't want her to see me in such a state, such a place. It was more palatable for me when we hiked two miles only a week after my release.

But my release had yet to come, and I remained in the hospital with a plastic tube up my nose. (How did they force food up my nose anyway?) Clearly, the hospital had a protocol, not always individualized, and for the next week, or so, I tried to figure it out.

Why was I being checked for bed sores?

"I'm hardly ever in bed," I said.

"Yes," the bed sore checker said, "but we're required to check. You'd be surprised at how many people lie in bed all day long."

"Really? That would drive me insane."

Every day someone came in and squeezed my belly skin into a bunch and stabbed me with a thumbtack. Of course it was a sterilized needle, but it sure looked and felt like a tack. "What's that for?" I asked.

"It's to prevent you from getting blood clots."

"Why would I get blood clots?"

"From lying around in bed all day."

One young helper was so chipper with her high-pitched happy voice that she seemed a caricature of the "candy-stripe" hospital helper, perky boobs, thin waist, ultra-blonde hair. Before I became a patient, I might have merely found her irritating, but under the circumstances she was surprisingly welcome, and I now understand the value of her unbounded enthusiasm. How else to approach such a job? I enjoyed her bobbing around and helping. One patient, a thin smoker with long tangled hair and tubes taped to her face, screamed at the helper so much that she told the nurses. "I'm sorry, I need help with that patient." She explained about being yelled at and demeaned. Then added, "She said that I would not pneumonia her any more." Nobody knew what that meant but the intent seemed mean.

I was returning from one of my walks, leaned close to the happy helper, and managed to enunciate through my bandages, "For what it's worth," I said, "I don't think you've pneumonia-ed anybody."

Her high perky laugh echoed in the hall, and I thought she might have an overabundance of estrogen, which reminded me again of the overabundance of stuff I know nothing about, my admiration for these doctors, nurses, and other medical professionals increasing just as much as my desire to get away from them.

I would love to identify each nurse by name, outline their courageous, positive characteristics, but nurses rotate shifts, and their shifting faces blended together with each caring attitude replaced by another, slightly different but no less dedicated and professional. They were all warm and cheerful under dire circumstances, caregivers worth every bit of hyperbole I could pile on. Considering what they do, they, like teachers, are underpaid. I often thanked them, and enjoyed my relationship with each of them. Even April, for without April how could I be a May, and if that makes sense to you, then you might want to consider therapy, or writing, or both.

Aside from the mini, mostly useless TVs in each room, a full sized TV was in the waiting area near the elevator next to the best window for viewing Forest Park. On rare occasions, mostly at night, I stood and watched TV for a few minutes. The TV was perpetually on, annoyingly, without anyone watching it, blasting detergent commercials at midnight. I always turned it off. Aside from being TV-depressing, wasn't it wasting electricity? So I was being nobly and altruistically productive, right? Somehow, regardless of the rationale, turning off that TV made me feel better.

One woman had wheeled her room's oversized lounge chair into the waiting area, set it up directly in front of the TV, blocking the window and monopolizing the TV, occasionally falling asleep. Once, I turned it off while she was sleeping and wheeled away fast. When I returned she scowled at me.

For a long time, a Latino woman sat in the waiting room, overwrought, speaking into her cellphone. "Yes, of course I love you. Don't you want me to help. No, don't say that. I do love you. I do." And so on endlessly, day after day. I assumed she was speaking to her dying-of-cancer husband. Isn't that what this sixth floor was all about? Dying or mutilated cancer patients? I'd seen many with holes in their throats.

I wheeled past a room, a mother and father telling their daughter that the tests showed cancer. I heard the wailing and weeping. I saw the relatives coming and going, and the doctors and therapists. I watched the drama of the sixth floor because I was rarely in my room. Were all the others watching me when I wept with the therapist Shannon Nana?

According to Kim, the nurses had begun to call me their "star walker." Obviously, they weren't fans of "The Walking Dead." Or maybe they were and they thought I looked like a zombie. Once, I was joined by a walker who was by no means a zombie. He was round and soft, holding his IV pole like a stand-up microphone, skipping and dancing up and down the halls. He had on big headphones connected to his Ipod. (Too bad we no longer use walkmans; I bemoan the loss of bad puns because of new technology.) After three days, the round man disappeared, maybe dancing his way to heaven? Or hell? Or back to the operating table? Or a "special" floor, something more secure than the sixth floor? I don't know. Maybe he was now healthily dancing his way down the city streets. But I admired his attitude. Dance! We should all dance like that. Or maybe not. My step by slow step mirrored my slogs up mountains. His obviously reflected a different life. And my questioning his life shows more about me than it does him. He's likely with loved ones now, singing on holidays, maybe dancing on a stage somewhere.

There were other walkers. The sixth floor smokers. I had a rare salivary gland cancer not attributable to smoking. Theirs was throat cancer directly attributable to smoking. One guy mouthed that it was "quiet time." I wondered if his quiet time would be for the rest of his life. Mine would not be. For a moment, I felt superior. Ha! I made it and you didn't. It was a savage competition for "quality of life." I won. You didn't. But holy crap what an empty thought! Fleeting, fortunately. Was it a "normal" feeling of competition? I'd rather be playing soccer with them, kicking a ball past their goal post, not sharing a quiet nod or a knowing glance in the sixth floor hallway.

I felt bad for them. But I also felt that I wasn't one of them. They had it worse. I had made it through. Obviously, I could talk, and I could swallow, even though continual greenish-brown phlegm oozed from my mouth. But Kim told me that the operation had gone well, that preliminary results were good. I don't know about these others, but I was just passing through. Where would their trip lead them? If I thought about it too much, it might break my heart. I couldn't absorb any more, I couldn't. I needed to be selfish.

Curiously, two Latino young men arrived in the waiting room, also talking on their cellphones, making jokes, some in Spanish, and I could understand a few words. Then on my walk around the corner and down the lead-nurse side of the dirty carpeted hall, I glanced into a room and saw the Latino woman sitting next to someone with a massive brace, long screws into the skull. It became clear, or as clear as anything could be in this odd reality, that the woman's son had broken his neck. I figured a bicycle accident, or motorcycle, or falling from a roof. What was he doing here? With all us cancer patients? The young man looked as if he would recover. Was he paralyzed? I didn't know. But for some reason, I thought not. He was young. He would recover. He was fine, and he would live a long healthy life. That's what I thought then and what I choose to believe now, regardless of how wrong I could be. Whenever possible, I choose, perhaps fatalistically, to remain optimistic. And while "fatal optimism" may seem like an oxymoron, that's how my thoughts progressed in this bizzaro world.

While I was able to sleep, saved by my wife, Lynn, Shannon Nana, Doctor Clarke, and others, I was still interrupted continually. My new concoction of antibiotics took longer to drip. Sitting and staring at the fluids dripping was deadly dull, and the nurses wouldn't let me lie down. "You might aspirate." So I walked even more than before.

One night, late, just as I finished the antibiotic drip and my sleep-inducing Percocet, a nurse said it was feeding time. I had to finish my feed bag before I could go to sleep. That meant another hour. I was exhausted. I had just climbed to 18,000 feet and wanted the slumber of base camp, and now they were telling me that I had to return to the summit for dinner.

By now, I had learned how to feed. Hook the syringe up to the nose tube. Pull back until you get backwash, usually a disagreeable discharge from your stomach. If the backwash stops at a certain point on the syringe, then you "eat." The backwash step seemed unnecessary. It was feeding time. If there was anything we know how to do, it's how to overeat. I measured exactly, down to the milliliter, the amount of liquid "food," hospital-grade industrial-strength energy drink, basically high-priced Ensure, and I poured it in the feed bag, then hooked it up to the tube. After the food was gone, you "flushed" the tube with an exact amount of water. Got it. Mostly, I had the nurses do it because if you screwed up a step, fluids sprayed, dripped, or oozed everywhere.

But I volunteered to do it on my own. "I need the practice."

Then, when they weren't looking, I steered myself back into my room, clanged the metal pole into the tiny bathroom, and dumped liquid food into the toilet. I carefully measured the water by eyeballing it, flushed the tube, and announced I was ready for bed.

After that incident, I took control of my schedule, arranging to have my pain medication, my vitals checked, my antibiotics, and my feeding at the same time, shifting them an hour one way or the other, thus allowing me a full four or five hours without interruption. Then, if I was roused for mysterious reasons in the middle of the night, I could take an Ambien and sleep the rest of the way.

During the final resort days, a male nurse who I nicknamed Sheldon after the character from TV's "The Big

Bang Theory" had trouble finding a workable IV port in my pincushion arms. He tried once, twice, three times, went away, and came back to try a fourth time, sweat visible on his brow. Finally, I just told him that it was okay to ask for help. Both he and I were too tense to get it done. I could smell the cigarette smoke sweating out of him. He was one of many nurses who wandered out of the building on their break and smoked. Funny how they can disconnect themselves from the damaged smokers, those with gaping holes in their throats.

Another nurse came in and had some trouble but was finally able to establish the port in my arm, the only vein left willing to accept the intrusion.

A release date was drawing near. I could feel it. I asked about it daily. I also cautiously asked a nurse about "the noise," the low-level whispering sound.

"Do you hear something?" I asked. "Music maybe."

She paused, cocked her head. "No, don't hear anything."

I would have pursued it further, but feared they might want to keep me longer, for further evaluation. While I will never know where it came from, I do know that the odd noise seeping into my room was real, not my imagination or drug-induced hallucination. Haven't heard it since. Aliens? Maybe. Seemed rational to blame it on the 1980s disco default music video. That's what I'm sticking to. So don't ask me about it.

A radiologist appeared, and we discussed exchanging my nose tube for a stomach feeding tube. It sounded great, another step to my release, but it also entailed local anesthesia and a "simple" procedure that punctured a hole through my stomach muscles. Interesting. My psyche bent to the memory of my hallucinogenic post-op ordeal.

My current daytime nurse was celebrating her last day before retiring. She was an efficient nurse who was enamored of procedure, and she was determined to make sure Kim and I knew the feeding procedure so we could perform it properly at home. It didn't matter of course that everyone – nurses, dieticians, doctors, cleaning personnel – taught the feeding procedure. Never mind that I had been "feeding" myself for the past couple days. Never mind that I was sick to death of it. But the retiring nurse insisted that we needed to watch a video about the procedure. She spoke in slow upper Midwest vernacular.

I was jumping out of my skin with terror about my stomach drilling operation. My body reacted viscerally as if another 12-hour assault were about to begin. Yet, here we stood watching the miniature TV on the mechanical arm going over every detail about the feeding bag, the measuring cup, the syringe. The person in the video was a younger version of the retiring nurse, a person who had dedicated her life to helping others and who had embraced hospital protocol as the surest way to success. Her delivery in the video was even more ponderous than her nearly identical real life explanations about how to feed at home. Monstrous insects were burrowing through my body searching for my brain.

The video ended, thank God, and the nurse began discussing it with us. Kim was chatty and polite. She didn't know about my monster insects. Finally, I interrupted. "I'm sorry, but please could I have some time alone with my wife. I know how to feed myself. We've been over it a 100 times. I have an operation tomorrow and I'm terrified. I just need to talk to my wife."

I thought I was being polite enough. But maybe not. The nurse looked startled. Maybe she even flashed a Nurse Ratchet smile. Or maybe that was my imagination. She left, never to be seen again. Retired. Everybody on the sixth floor disappeared, presumably somewhere eating cake.

I looked at Kim. "Her video," I said, "made me want to rip my eyes out."

Then I launched into my fear about the tube in my stomach operation. It may have been irrational, but I was terrified. And since when is terror rational? I didn't want to go anywhere near an operating table. What if something went wrong? What if I ended up in a room with April? She was gone. Or was she? Maybe she was lurking in the dark hallways.

The procedure was scheduled for 11 and would only

take about a half-hour. So at 10:30 they came for me. I asked the attendant with the wheel-away bed if I could walk, but a raspy voiced (obvious smoker) nurse technician told him not to allow it, he could lose his job. So I climbed on the bed and rode it around corners, down the elevator, down a hall, onto another elevator, eventually to an area where I was moved to a waiting bed, lined up with others in more dire shape, where I waited. I sat up. I peered around the curtain. I watched a big guy lean heavily into an attractive technician and heard him say, "Hey baby, what about it? I been asking you for months so let's get it on tonight." Had to be a joke, I thought. If not, his continued heavy handed advances were the worst and most obvious form of sexual harassment I'd ever witnessed. Maybe to stop it I tried to get his attention. I was able to corral him and ask him why it was taking so long, in a nice way of course. He said he'd see what he could do. I overheard him talking to another tech. "That's a big name for down here." They were referring to my surgeon, Doctor Haughey.

Soon after, I was wheeled past others into a room where I was lifted onto a metal table with a round mechanical technical device above me. There were several of these rooms arranged like spokes around the waiting area, and people were wheeled in and out, a regular assembly line.

Before I knew what was going on, the drill came spinning fast down into me. And then out. Like I was a two-by-four at a construction site. I felt nothing. And they said I was done, my anxiety gone in a puff of sawdust.

I was zooming around the curves and corridors back to my sixth floor room where I was able to stand and resume my walking, now with a tube hanging from my stomach, and my nose. Not long after, a doctor showed up to remove the nose tube. No procedure, no anesthetic, nothing really. He sat down in front of me, told me to hold still, gripped the tube and pulled. That was it. Stomach tube in. Nose tube out.

Okay, I thought, let's go home.

The next day, Friday May 4, I was going to be discharged. Kim sent me a text message. "A few more hours. We can make it because we're a team. Get some sleep so you heal fast."

Discharge day is of course anxiety inducing and exciting. Would I have to stay another day? When exactly could I leave?

"I love you! Can't wait to have you home. Kimberly."

I changed into street clothes. The psychiatrist Doctor Clarke came by to see how I was faring. "Fine," I said, "Thanks. You are a smart guy." I met with doctors, technicians, dieticians, and Lynn. Kim arrived in my room and despite making idle conversation, I still wasn't out of the hospital. I walked Lynn out. We were saying goodbye outside when Kim called and said that Doctor Haughey was in my room waiting for me. By the time I got back, he'd left, and we had to wait longer for my discharge. (Coincidentally, I was talking to Lynn on my cellphone when we missed our appointment time in Philadelphia.)

Eventually Doctor Haughey returned. I sat in the 1980s lounge chair and he sat next to me, surrounded by his crew. He touched my arm and said, "We got it out with clear margins all around."

"Thank you," Kim said.

"Thank you," I said.

"No reason to thank me," he responded, "I was just doing my job."

"Okay," I said, "thanks for not screwing it up."

He seemed to like that one.

"Unfortunately," he said, "You will require radiation." He looked disappointed having to recommend radiation, but since the tumor had invaded a nerve, it was required to make sure it didn't come back.

"What about chemotherapy?" Kim asked.

No chemotherapy (no Doctor Wilde).

Still glowing from the idea of clear margins, and no chemo, we shrugged off radiation. After all, we'd faced the inevitability of radiation. No big deal. We were going to beat this. What was a little radiation? (What did we know?) We shook hands, and Doctor Haughey left, followed by his crew.

We waited for the discharge papers, suffering more questions, and instructions. "I do not," I said to everyone who would listen, "under any circumstances, need instruction about feeding."

I waited for someone to remove the bandages, only slightly disappointed to hear that I would need to keep them for two weeks. Kim and I took our discharge papers and I left my IV pole behind, thanked the nurses, waved goodbye, took one last walk down the long hallway with the shiny wood floors, and left the hospital, a POW shuffling through the gates of freedom.

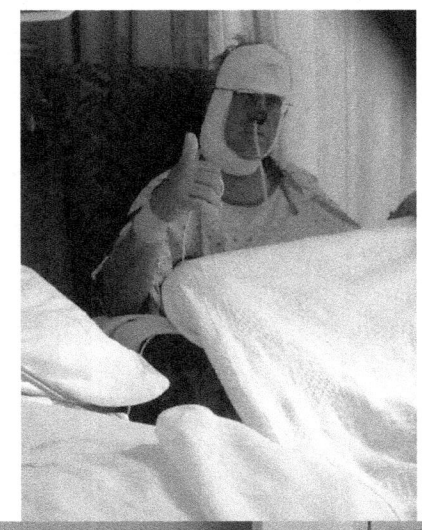

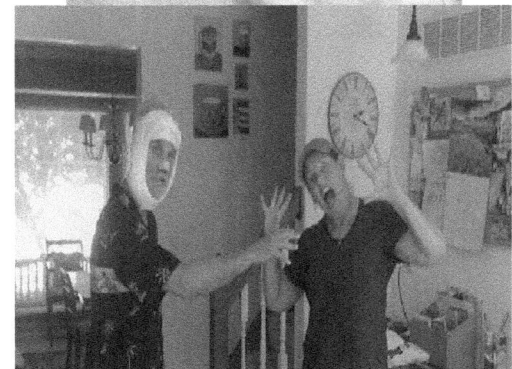

Escaping the Bizarre: Hospital to Home

Chapter Twenty – Home in May

Kim drove, gliding on air, the highway smooth, spring
sunlight through the windshield, heading toward home and
the promise of uninterrupted sleep and normalcy. That is, if
it was normal to have bandages wrapped tight around my
head, tube dangling from my stomach, swollen tongue and
foul mouth. Who's to say what's normal, right? Compared to
my cellmates at the hospital, I was a pillar of strength and
energy.

Inside, a welcome home sign hung over the fireplace,
and balloons, Sarah ready with a hug and Sam releasing
himself from his computer to come downstairs and stand by
until I offered up a hug. Then onto the deck and the new
canopied and cushioned deck swing awaiting my first nap in
the balmy air.

While I passed out on the swing, Sarah tried to get my
fifteen complex prescriptions filled at COSTCO where
pharmacy protocol and the sparse supply of drugs left her
feeling inadequate, the pharmacist treating her like a dumb
teenager. Sarah, while she was still technically a teenager,
was anything but dumb. Of course, most of us say that about
our kids, so why would you believe me? But really, it's true.
Ask anybody. Frustrated, she returned with only two of the
medications. The others, the pharmacist insisted, might be
ready on Monday.

Dave Lancaster walked down and was talking with Kim
when I woke to prescription chaos. The list of medications
was daunting. Ambien, Cleocin, Docusate-senna,
Esomprazole, Nystatin, folic acid, flucoasole,
Acetaminophen liquid, Oxycodone, Lexapro and five or six
more. Most of them prescribed in liquid form. We tried to

figure it out. Sarah felt like she had failed us. After reassuring her, we continued deciphering the medications. Ambien. That was for sleeping, but for now I knew how to sleep – just pass out on the new deck swing. Kim and Sarah bought it specifically for my napping. Cleocin "for treating bacteria in the vagina." What? Did I now have a vagina? Did they replace my tongue with a... no wonder they always asked your name, birthday, and procedure. Apparently, upon further reading, we found that Cleocin is used to treat bacterial infections in the mouth and since I still had a yellow swirl of phlegm, I needed Cleocin.

Docusate, a stool softener, and Senna was a laxative that would allow me to... (sorry, I almost insulted my reader with stating the obvious and nobody deserves that shit). Did I need a stool softener for the weekend? John Zavgren, during his crushed arm ordeal, made the hyperbolic statement that he had "the worst case of constipation known to humankind." Near the end of my hospital stay, I had yet to crap, and I was worried they wouldn't set me free until I had a bowel discharge. I considered lying. Presumably with the help of docusate-senna, I did it. And I found the nearest doctor, leaned close to her and proudly announced my stupendous achievement. But did I absolutely need docusate-senna now, during my first couple nights at home? Next was the Esomeprazole for heartburn. No, probably didn't need that unless the chaos continued.

And it did. I was pacing around the kitchen table as evening descended. Dave and Kim chatted about what I considered insignificant suburban travails. We still did not have my medicine. I was sure that one of these medicines, unless I had it, would boomerang me back into the hospital.

The following sequence was another of my dark moments. I could have acted differently I suppose, but I think we assumed that upon returning home, most of my problems would dissolve into a safe routine.

I slammed my fist on the kitchen table. "Give me the Goddamn prescriptions. I'll drive over and get them filled."

"Come on Jeff," Dave said, "You don't want to do that."

No, I didn't, of course, and it probably would have been

a disaster. I would have passed out between the protein bars and Raisinets. But faced with wobbling and staggering alone through the bright lights of a super-discount store and returning to the hospital, I was ready to take my chances.

"Nobody else will." I grabbed my car keys.

"No," Kim shouted. "Don't do this!"

Was this a scene from bad TV, from USA network or Lifetime? If so, hopefully something enlightening like Swamp Hog Hunters. Kim called COSTCO, talked to the pharmacist and despite her extraordinary efforts, got nowhere.

Sam stumbled down from his room. "What's going on?"

Dave was exhausted after working all day and now he was being entwined in family drama, more than he had bargained for, having come down to "celebrate."

"Call me if I can help," he said, fleeing up the street.

I withdrew to our TV room where I could watch actors play out silly scenes like ours. Kim, Sam, and Sarah began the slow process of piecing together what medicine was absolutely needed, where we could get it, and from whom. Psychiatrist Lynn called in two prescriptions. Sarah and Sam picked up vitamins, over-the-counter substitutes, and prescription medicine from Walgreens and a return trip to COSTCO. Sam came into the TV-room where I was bleary-eyed and vacantly staring at TV nonsense, feed bag hooked up to my stomach tube. He said, "I know you feel bad, but we can take care of you okay. You've taken care of us, now it's our turn." He hugged me. With the help of my family, I would remain out of the hospital, free.

In the morning, around nine, I walked down our neighborhood street around the cul-de-sac. Not very far, shorter than some of my hospital walks, but a walk nonetheless, and I was outside in the fresh, suburban air. But I was also still in lots of pain, mainly in my shoulder and back. And I was still disconnected from the world, my head wrapped tight, a zombie nodding at neighbors walking their dogs.

A feeding pole and a box of feeding bags arrived on our front porch, the pole a rental, and the bags a $500 contested cost even though we were told they would be covered. Kim tried to hook up the big syringe to my tube, measure out the backwash, mix medications into the liquid, all with me telling her what to do, how to do it, and when she did something wrong. It didn't take very long for us to come to an understanding. I should take care of myself, my feedings and when to take meds. I felt more in control of my own fate, and she obviously had no desire to listen to me crab at her.

I followed my schedule, measuring out exactly the amount I was supposed to take, pouring it into the bag, attaching it to the tube, and sitting. Forever, it seemed. I skipped checking the backwash. And soon it became apparent that the pole was more or less superfluous. I used it only in the TV room, but could have easily arranged something. In my office, I attached the bag to the wall while I meditated. I moved it to the other wall while I worked on my computer. I carried it with me when I had to pee. I held it high while I smiled in the mirror at my scraggly self staring back at me. Merely the act of smiling improves your mood. Sometimes it doesn't work so well. In my final year as Associate Director at Metropolitan School, during my 20-munite morning commute, I put a pen between my teeth so that I would be forced to smile the whole way. When I entered, a few teachers gathered around me, gawking. "Are you okay," they asked.

"Sure, why?"

They told me to look in the mirror. My lips were nothing but blue ink.

Now at home, I took a mirror picture of myself. Not that I wouldn't remember, but I was seeking cancer comedy, and I sort of looked funny. In a hurry to get back to my office and my keyboard, I turned as if my next Twitter comment would change history, only to have my tube catch on the bathroom cabinet handle.

Holy crap! My guts ripped out! Stopping me fast. I pulled up my T-shirt expecting to see blood. My skin was stretched, the stitches still holding the tube in place, but dangling just a bit lower. After many more yanks, catching the tube on kitchen handles, forgetting to disconnect from the pole or the wall, stepping on the tube while hurrying upstairs, I was pretty sure it wouldn't come out unless I purposely yanked and pulled. But it never felt good.

I still wasn't supposed to talk too much, so I emailed a lot. It was gratifying to write that the tumor was out with clear margins, but I felt overwhelmed by looming financial burdens and had another dark moment, desperately trying to regain $65,000 dollars worth of control over my life. I emailed, "Your welshing at this point almost seems cruel to me."

When Kim asked me simple unrelated questions, I often responded with irritated one-word answers. I wrote her a note, apologizing for being grouchy, "When people have expectations about how I should respond, I am forced to grunt. Don't mind being a caveman, but I get no caveman privileges... no hunting with clubs. Love you lots. You saved my life. Your husband, life partner, lover, and best friend."

By Monday, May 7, a few days removed from the hospital, I started writing this book, my Cancer Comedy, writing one thought, one line at a time, then napping. My feeding and medicine schedule consumed big portions of my day. I loved reading and napping on the deck swing.

I watched TV and videos, and was particularly bothered by the TV ads with the hot skinny chicks opening their mouths big and wide to bite into a massive triple-beef, bacon-cheeseburger, loaded with condiments. Eating like that will make you fat, could give you cancer, and has little to do with sex.

I spoke to Jim on the phone, apparently at a time of heightened lucidity for me.

He emailed, "You sounded remarkably well. Did you ever hear that Churchill quote? The one that advises: 'If you're going through hell keep going'."

I told him I was reading Great Plains, and he suggested I should be reading "Great Pains." I sent him the picture of me in the bathroom mirror. He responded by referencing trout.

"I prefer the ones stuck to my office wall: you holding the big brown while standing in the bone-numbing cold water of Spring Creek, the photo of you with John holding a damn nice rainbow after two geniuses shattered your van window...."

Andi Boyd visited with John Reichle, and she sat next to me on the swing, mostly talking to Kim while I listened. Listening was much easier than talking. But also disturbing. When my friend Bob, Claire's husband, slipped into his decade-long illness and nursing home stay, he more or less stopped talking. When people stop talking, they enter a different reality and since I've spent much of my life as a writer in varying silent realities, I feared that I could all too easily give up talking and become a nonentity, like my friend Bob in the nursing home. And I recalled an episode of "The Twilight Zone" in which a notoriously verbose individual made a bet that he could go one year without uttering a word, but at the end of the year, he'd lost his ability to talk.

However, listening to Andi sitting next to me on the swing was much better than allowing my mind to fast forward 30 years, as I had been doing, imagining myself sitting silently on the edge of a far away cliff waiting to die. (Hmm, somehow that image doesn't strike me as very funny.)

On May 9, Julie texted asking if she should visit, and I responded, "Okay, but no running yet, and talking limited."

"No worries, I talk enough for two ... or three or four people:)"

That was an exaggeration, of course. She does not, as her joke implies, monopolize conversations. Rather she's an excellent conversationalist, the right balance of listening and speaking. Uncharacteristically, however, she showed up in flip-flops, expecting me to shuffle down the street like most people just a week removed from the hospital. I suggested she needed better shoes. She borrowed a pair from Kim, and we hiked a couple miles at Forest 44 Conservation Area where few people would see me bandaged up, not that either of us cared.

On May 8, Kim and I went in to have the bandage changed. The moments without the wrap felt liberating. But tightly, back on, it went and I swear that's the last you'll hear a Yoda imitation. But I can't promise I won't force a bad metaphor or two; for example, my head felt like a black bean burrito wrap, the kind of meal I would have trouble swallowing.

We went to see the swallow doctor, Archie Harmon. He felt that I had a "very good chance."

"Even after radiation?" I asked.

"That will make it more difficult."

"But I will be able to swallow, right?"

"Right," he said, businesslike, not very enthusiastically.

By Monday, May 14, I was walking in the woods two miles almost every day, but after every walk I fell asleep, the fatigue wearing on my psyche. And I discovered that I couldn't pucker. A simple sign of affection, the pucker kiss. I kept pressing my lips to Kim and felt nothing. She said I felt fine, but from my side, my lips felt like a limp handshake. I couldn't drink from a straw either, so I became obsessed with milkshakes and kissing Kim.

I emailed my indispensable psychiatrist friend, Lynn. "Was three weeks to suck and pucker asking too much?" But she was still struggling with her hip replacement, so we analyzed each other and concluded that we were both screwed.

I wrote, "When are you going to come sit on the deck with me in the sun and talk about what sucks and then rebuild our perspectives into positive outlooks? You will get better and you will be able to walk and ride in canoes and sit in the water while I fish. It will take time. Took Zavgren six months. I'm sure we both can heal sooner than that... geez... all he did was crush his arm."

Zavgren was cutting down a tree next to the gushing creek and waterfall in his New Hampshire "yard," when it "unexpectedly" fell the wrong way, landing on his arm, crushing it. Now he was calling me, checking on me, and we talked about recovery. I told him I felt bad about his arm, not even knowing anything about it until my son Sam and I went to visit him in 2009. He had been unable to hike with us and was still taking pain killers. The doctors had wanted to cut his arm off. They told him that in a year it would just be flopping about and would just get in the way. He declined.

Now, while not as strong as it once was, he has full use of his arm. Zavgren talked to me a lot before my big operation – encouraging to hear about his recovery when I was facing loss of my tongue. Like his arm, I would not let them chop off my tongue.

Jim emailed, "Who said life was supposed to be fun? I wonder if it's a 50/50 split between fun and unfun? Then, contemplating this, if you think about the plight of the other peoples of this planet, you sure can feel like a self-centered jerk, can't you?"

We had discussed this before. While I also had selfish reasons, the plight of others compelled me to stay at Metropolitan School for 15 years. Despite my anxieties, I enjoyed life and couldn't figure out why the world had to suffer so much.

By May 15, I had a nice breakthrough – with lots of practice, I was able to drink a cup of coffee and eat a bowl of fruit. Then we went back to Archie the swallow doctor, and he shoved paste in my mouth and told me to swallow it while he watched with his x-ray vision machine. Unfortunately, he said that lots of the "food" was going nowhere, just sitting on my windpipe. I would have to limit my swallowing to three bites a day of Jello or pudding. I hate pudding. Jello is worse.

On May 19, I was liberated from my bandages and my tongue didn't fall apart. And now I could wash my hair, stand in the shower and let the warm water splatter and run down my shoulders, having to shout at myself, "Get out!" Otherwise, my skin would dry like a molting snake in the sun. I reveled in the freedom of my head in the cool spring air, and hiked at various times with Claire, Julie, Dave Lancaster, Kim, my brother John, and on my own. I kept moving because without movement there would be no healing. I needed to be strong to withstand the next onslaught. Radiation.

Kim and I visited the radiologist, but Doctor Gay was out of town for several weeks. The replacement doctor, a white-coat with glasses, someone who assumed authority with ease, started describing the radiation process, 69 "grays" on the right side.

Kim seemed to understand what the hell he was talking about. "That seems like a lot," she said.

"Yes, it's a little high, but based on the clinical studies, it's most effective for this type of cancer." He waited, apparently for more questions, then continued, "But much less, 35, on the left side."

"Wait and minute!" I said, "No one said we had to do both sides! It's on the right, why do we need to radiate the left?"

"We were," Kim said, "under the impression that we would only need to radiate the left side. Now you're saying both sides. How will this affect his swallowing?"

"Well, obviously that will decrease his chances of swallowing."

"How much?"

"About ten to fifteen percent."

"So," I said, "You're saying that I have to radiate my left side as well, and my chances of being able to swallow go from one hundred to maybe eighty-five?"

"Yes."

"So," I said, "there's a chance I won't be able to swallow... at all?"

"Yes."

"That's not acceptable," Kim said. "We're all about quality of life."

Hearing that phrase again nearly sent me to the parking lot. "Stop," I muttered. "We're fine. If that's what it takes, we'll do it."

Kim, brilliantly ignoring me, pressed on. "There are always other options. What are they?"

"Well, I almost hesitate to bring this up, but..."

"What?" Kim asked.

"There is a test trial."

"What is it?"

"We could do a neck dissection on the unaffected side and if it's clear of cancer, we wouldn't need to radiate that side."

"How does that affect swallowing?"

"We haven't done that many, so there aren't a lot of

clinical trials."

"Okay," Kim asked, "but what are the odds?"

"Well so far, with only a few trials, one-hundred percent positive."

"You mean, one-hundred percent able to swallow?"

"Yes. But even if the left side is clear, you could have long-term radiation damage. It's just that your odds are much better."

Kim and I looked at each other and knew immediately that we would choose the test trial. What would you have done?

"We'll need," the radiologist said, "to make sure Doctor Haughey approves."

"He will," Kim said.

I knew of course that Kim had saved me again, but I hated the idea of returning to the hospital for another surgery even though we were well into May and April wasn't there anymore. But what would May bring? (These useless puns are my revenge for being called April and June in grade school.) Would this surgery be another marathon into hell, a hallucinatory experience hurling me into a three-week hospital abyss?

No use thinking about it too much. I needed to heal as much as I could so they could cut me open again, my third surgery scheduled for May 24, a week away. And I had to look "normal" when we closed on our home refinance.

After months of delay, First Community Credit Union sent a final settlement statement, showing an increased interest rate and thousands due at closing on the day after surgery. In another spate of intensive phone conversations, Kim asked pointed questions about rolling the cash due into the loan and about the rate. The processor said, "We had additional costs that made the rate go up to four percent."

"No," Kim said, "We agreed to 3.875. With twenty percent down, it's a win-win for you guys."

They reset the rate, rolled in the cash, and changed the closing date to May 29, giving me three days for recovery before I'd have to fake sincerity, act normal, and sign dozens of legal documents.

Naturally, during this mortgage process, I felt compelled to email John Toppen. Before the Great Recession, we joked about him being a real estate "Guru," but after, he referred to himself as the "No-Good-Brother-In-Law."

> Admittedly, my last email was from the edge. I'm starting to feel a little better, but I'm still on that edge. Everyone has been phenomenal in their belief in my full recovery. I have the same belief in you. You will recover from this mess that you're in and inescapably, the mess my family and I are also in. Probably don't have to remind you, but so much of our life's work and effort hinges on your success now. I wish I could just tell you to forget about it. No big deal, I've sold a billion copies of my books, and repayment can come whenever, but I can't. We are in no position to do so. And at some point our kids will want to go back to college, and we will have to tell them there's no money to help them with that. We will barely have enough to cover our health insurance, food, gas, and so on, and our life savings will start draining away even more. I don't expect to be able to work again until January 2013. I know you can pull through this. It will be difficult. But it can be done.

His response alluded to a cheap paperback Garth Brooks biography that we surreptitiously exchanged for years, hiding it in each others luggage, sending it as a birthday or Christmas gift, sharing our disdain for "modern" country music. "I know what the bill is. My urine sample is on it's way. Maybe we should both coauthor a book on human misery and other insightful musings. You are well on your way to full recovery. Hang in there. We will both make it. I will treat you to a Garth Brooks concert when you have fully recovered."

Also, in the days prior to my third surgery (fourth if you counted the biopsy) and the refinance, Kim's medical leave of absence was expiring. Rather than seek an extension for the last few days of school, she decided to go back, work with the substitute, end on a positive note, and clear out her belonging. Unfortunately, her boss saw this as an opportunity for retaliation, maintaining stone-silent distance while manipulating the substitute, making it extremely difficult to transition from teaching to early retirement. What should have been a joyous retirement year celebrating 25 years of dedication, felt more like a dismissal, a brush back, a good riddance. Instead of retiring with dignity, the boss made sure it was anything but a celebratory occasion, successfully creating a hostile working environment not only for Kim, but for others and, given the opportunity, would do so in the future. (After a year of appropriate scrutiny, in early 2013, the principal-boss was forced into early retirement.)

Chapter Twenty-One – The Third Op

On Thursday, May 24, one week removed from our radiologist visit and our decision to have test trial surgery, I was on the operating table again. Given Doctor Haughey's attention and professionalism, the fast action wasn't surprising, but we weren't prepared for the extent of the surgery. It was not a simple Doctor Fred neck dissection. This time Doctor Haughey took out about 60 lymph nodes, and it knocked me on my ass. "You'll be fine Jeff:)"

The morning after my surgery, I was lying in a much more comfortable hospital bed than my previous incarceration. But the doctors then explained that I would have to stay in the hospital for a few days, maybe up to a week because they had to monitor my fluids for something Kim said was called KIAs, but that seems more like a car, or Killed In Action. I still don't understand what it was. Sure, the bed was comfortable, but no way I wanted to stay in it for a week.

"I want to go home," I said, likely sounding like an exhausted, whiney little kid at an amusement park. Maybe my whining worked. Or maybe Doctor Haughey just knew me well enough to know that I'd be better off at home. He came in about an hour later and told me I could go that day.

"Great!" Then I added, looking for reassurance, "This was a good choice, wasn't it?"

"We'll have to wait for the test results," he said, "but I didn't see much of anything…."

I gave him a thumbs up, then said, "I feel like I got into a fight. I brought my boxing gloves and the other guy brought a switchblade."

Of course I used this line over and over again for the

next month and only got a smattering of a chuckles. Probably because it sounds like I stole it from a bad B movie. In my defense, it did accurately reflect my feelings.

We would need to keep the drainage tube in for a week, monitoring the amount, color, and consistency of the fluids. If the fluid was murky, we would need to call. If there was too much, we would need to call. If the tube popped out, blood squirting across the floor... call for help.

Kim sprang me from the hospital a day after surgery, and I was home again. Immediately, I walked down the street and around the cul-de-sac, Sarah telling me to "take it easy."

I said, "This is me taking it easy."

But that evening my bravado faded quickly when I started shaking uncontrollably and my left side turned red. I crawled into bed hoping I hadn't taken it so "easy" that I'd end up back in the hospital. Like the other surgeries, I had a neck drainage tube, but unlike the others, my left shoulder was tender and tingly numb, and I could barely lift my head. My neck from ear to ear ached and it felt like someone was strangling me. (Now, as I write this in October, after radiation, that strangling feeling is tighter than ever, but I will recover.)

I was feeling down, worse than down, worse than the other surgeries.

Once again, friends and family responded. Lynn texted, "Got my fingers crossed about outcome."

Lisa: "Got to go home quickly – that was good. Happy anniversary. We met 34 years ago this weekend."

Andi Boyd: "You gotta be totally sick of this! This is one of those times when you just gotta relinquish control and let them work their miracle. I know it's tough. Crazy stuff you never expected. One step at a time, one healing at a time until suddenly one day it all clicks. You can do this!"

John Zavgren: "Hang in there!"

Julie texted, "Hope you'll be up for a hike soon:)." I told her that I should probably lie low and that people were likely getting sick of me being sick, and being such a downer. She responded, "Don't be ridiculous! I always enjoy you:)"

Jim emailed, "How was your encounter with space aliens?"

"I'm ready to give in..."

He answered with the following:

> Bullshit. So you would rather stay in hell? Your five-word message is extremely counterproductive. You're going through excruciating things right now but you are on the right path and will get through it. You are not alone. So many people are praying for you it would stun you. So many of these people have had sad, horrible things happen to them and to their children, it would stun you. Yet they are not bitter and continue to reach out to those of us who are hurting, who are bleeding — like you. You are the antithesis of quit, Jeff. I know that you'll get through this. You will get through this just fine. You'll see. Jeff, you are going to make it; you are tough as nails and you will say to your illness, 'Fuck off. Get the f— off my back!' and it'll get off for good.

With two tubes in me, three slashes to my neck, and lots of medication, I was measuring my time by surgery dates and doctor visits and I suppose, judging from my parents, both in their nineties, that all your friends at some point turn into young doctors. It was too soon for me however because I was only 58 and if I can still calculate properly, I should have about 30 years before I truly become my parents. But I was not the same father to my daughter and son as my father was to me. There were similar characteristics of course but making statements simplifying generations of human progress often makes you sound like a simpleton – "My God, I've turned into my parents."

I wrote, "My expectations are to run a marathon when I'm 100." And other nonsense. At this critical juncture I was questioning the value of writing anything when I needed to write more than ever.

The afternoon of May 29, we finally closed on our refinance. My thick grey-white beard concealed one side of my neck but the other had been shaved clean for the third operation, a Charles Manson look, probably not too good for financial dealings. So I evened up, shaving carefully around my wounds. Then I dressed to conceal the tube jutting out the side of my neck and the frothy ball.

Kim and I sat across from our mortgage processor. Kim did the talking. We signed one paper after the other. Of course it wasn't a first home purchase or a first refinance, so we knew the drill. But for me signing the document verifying that our employment status had not changed felt unsettling. It was only one paper buried in the stack, but mentally I questioned it. Had our "status" changed? Could we have known what might happen? Would I be working? Would Kim ever teach again? We kept our mouths shut and signed. Our credit was outstanding. If we said anything, we might have to start the whole process over and re-qualify. Another three to six months. Sometimes absurdities need to be ignored.

Wednesday, May 30, was memorable because Lynn visited and we sat in the sun on the deck, sharing a beer. Although no doctor approved, or knew about it, I drank one whole beer through my mouth. I had to hold my breath during the swallows but I didn't choke. And the next day, June 1, the drainage tube carrying my frothy pink fluids was removed.

Claire and Thomas stopped by and chatted on the deck. I got a book from Thomas, *Safe from the Neighbors* written by his friend, fine literature, great writing and depressing as hell. I told Thomas that the author's photo gave the impression that he was an "ass from academia."

"He is arrogant," Thomas replied.

I have always been keenly aware of how obnoxious writers can be, especially when drunk, trying to push their latest "Great American Novel" upon unsuspecting friends and acquaintances. It's embarrassing, and I've written about it in articles and blogs with such titles as "Are you a Writer?" and "Are We All Great Writers?" My general discomfort about hawking my work didn't disappear with my illness. In fact, getting ill in itself seemed an embarrassment.

We got another one of those panic-inducing, test-result phone calls and for the first time during this ordeal, the result was welcome. All clear. None of the 60 nodes showed cancer. No need to radiate the left side.

Maybe in my subconscious I felt this was a turning point of some sort, a bit of good news that would swing the momentum back to my side and that would allow me to live, to hike, to fish, to grow old naturally. So I wrote an email on June 2 to a group of friends and family titled "My Cancer Comedy Update." I am writing this now at 10:30 PM, usually my bedtime, almost never a productive writing time for me. It's December 26, 2012, and apparently I've decided to include the entire email. If it survives the scrutiny of never ending revisions, then my initial logic has held up; that is, I rationalize including it here because even though partially repetitious, it will reflect the writing process, showing how I've used emails to piece together my broader narrative. Logic can be dangerous, I admit, allowing me to think I am breathing rare air while stupidly breaking literary rules I've embraced forever.

> This started out as an email and turned into drafting my book. So if you want to skip down to "Currently" for an update, I can hardly blame you. Not many want to read drafts of someone's crappy writing.

> If you're getting this email, I've already told you a lot, or you found out that I've been going through some health "difficulties" lately. I'm struggling to put the whole experience into a comedy format. You might understand that it is a struggle as there has been almost nothing funny about the whole trip other than the strange, weird, odd kind of funny. Nothing that would suggest comedy.

> But that's what I'm attempting because I have a habit of setting expectations so high and falling so short that the fall sometimes creates a chuckle or two. Just

as I write that though, I've already screwed up – I must believe in a full recovery or I will have little to no chance of a full recovery. But if I'm admitting to unrealistically high expectations, and always falling, then I've just undermined my recovery. See how funny it can get?

The mind games are endless. I walk a tightrope between needing to know and not wanting to know. For example, one radiologist was going to give me his spiel and a pamphlet about "what to expect" from the high doses of radiation. I said, "No thanks."

I already knew it wasn't going to be fun, that it is, in fact, going to be downright awful. No sense in dwelling on the particulars. I can compartmentalize my experience and have as much fun as possible learning to swallow prior to radiation so that I can lose that function during radiation and relearn it after. It is that sort of convoluted logic that sustains me. Only the essential information please. Half hour or so five days a week, five-ten minutes of actual radiation time. That's it. Don't want to know about the skin burns, the dry sore throat, the rubbery muscles, the... see? Who wants to think about that?

My descriptions of what happened are going to be false. But in essence they are true. It's just impossible for me to give a wholly accurate description. I'll do my best, though. So far, I've had a lovely time during a 12-hour surgery on April 23 at Barnes, waking to a hallucinogenic experience, sort of a bad LSD trip gone even more horribly wrong. The recovery "room" was a dungeon. No windows. Shadow creatures floating in and out while a brute of a nurse named April with spiked hair strapped me down, accused me of being an alcoholic, and stabbed me with needles. To be fair, I was screaming loudly and likely scaring others. But hell I thought I was in a real dungeon with April the master torture demon wielding long sharp needles while berating me, accusing me of having the DTs, of drinking way more than I reported. I could only scream, since I didn't know what was happening to me. Apparently, it was a reaction to twelve hours of anesthesia and to Cipro, a common antibiotic. If I would have known, I could have simply and calmly said to April, "Excuse me, nurse, my name is Jeffrey Penn May, born 12/27/1953 in here at Barnes for a neck dissection." They repeatedly ask you to tell them who you are and what your doing there to make sure they don't slit the wrong throat. "Excuse me, but I think I'm having a reaction to the antibiotic. April, I know we can work this out. Is there any chance we can convene a meeting of my surgical team now, at whatever late hour it is, on April 23, 2012?" That would have been the impossibly responsible thing to do. I afraid I acted poorly.

The anesthesia effects diminished, but it took over a week to figure out the reaction to Cipro. My legs would not stop shaking. My back hurt. I could not sit in a chair for more than a second. That's no exaggeration. I have witnesses.

This must be, I thought, how some of my students at Metropolitan School felt when I tried to teach them to at least "act normal." Granted, I did work hard to get their medication right, but they had a lot to deal with. More than I imagined back then. Was it a "failure of imagination?" Would we all be better off if we could imagine the souls of others? I don't know. Maybe. As long as we had control over it. It takes a special kind of person to imagine the plight of others, gain understanding, and effect positive change... without capitulating to the suffering, without having so much empathy that it overwhelms your own soul. Hmmm. That last bit didn't sound too funny. Maybe I'll need laugh tracks in this. Ha. Ha. You dumb shit, you're too empathetic. Ha. Ha.

Currently,

We went to the radiologist who said that we had a 10-15% chance of not being able to swallow because they would have to radiate both sides of my neck. Kim, who is absolutely brilliant, pressed the radiologist, telling him that wasn't acceptable. He hesitated, then mentioned a "test trial" whereby a neck dissection is done on the previously unaffected side and if it's clear of cancer, no need to radiate that side. Swallowing chances are almost 100% so far. What would you do? Of course we signed up and promptly, I was on the operating table again. This time they took out about 60 lymph nodes. The surgery knocked me on my ass for a few days. I had to have a drainage tube for a week, but we went to the doc yesterday and he took out the neck drainage tube, the staples, and thankfully told us that the lab report showed no cancer so no radiation on that side. In a few weeks, the final "treatment" phase will begin. I am very happy that my left side is okay. More or less. It has a three-inch slash. I brought my boxing gloves to a fight and the other guy showed up with his switchblade.

For the next few weeks I'm more or less available between appointments. Last Wednesday, May 30, a memorable date, Lynn Wakefield visited and we shared a beer. Although no doctor approved, or knows about it, I drank one whole beer through my mouth. I had to hold my breath during the swallows but I didn't choke. If you feel compelled to leave a review of one or more of my books, or purchase one or more of my books, I promise one choke-free swallow per purchase, and three choke-free swallows per review. I think I have this marketing business nailed.

Thank you for all your love and support.

The suggestion to buy my books was particularly embarrassing. On the other hand, for someone who was extremely cautious his entire life with using the word "love," my clichéd "thank-you-for-your-love" was surprisingly easy to write.

But what I am going to admit now, I know, will leave me open to all sorts of pop psychology interpretations about my character and personality, but my cancer ordeal, combined with the aging of my parents, finally allowed me to lower one last protective shield. For the first time I can remember, my mother said, straightforwardly, "I love you... too." The too added of course because I initiated it, saying it first, but perhaps I should have said it long before now, before my mother was showing signs of dementia, and before I was on the humorous side of cancer. Once, when I was leaving home to work on the Mississippi River towboats, she said, "Just remember, we still love you." But that was it more or less. Nothing stands out in my childhood except my mother getting angry at me for always needing stitches. What did she expect with two older brothers? And that was the crux of it. My mother suffered through four boys. She traveled on bumpy cargo planes across oceans with me as an infant clinging to her blouse and my brothers hanging onto her skirt. She holed up in remote bungalows while my spy father, having gone from WWII battlefields to secret passageways, disappeared for days at a time behind the Iron Curtain. She was the mother of rambunctious rowdy boys. So who could blame her for occasionally getting annoyed? Isn't it "funny" that cancer is a great tool for getting your Mom to say she loves you. I highly recommend it.

Even with their age-associated problems, my Mom and Dad retain a sharp sense of humor. We've joked about the travails of childrearing. And I recall a quote, "Raising kids is like being pecked to death by a duck."

Now I'm going to shift blame for this comedy to my

family and friends. Had they reacted to my email a little less enthusiastically, I might have decided against this impossible quest. So it's their fault.

Jim responded, "Much of your writing here has a crystalline hue, brilliance... no, you had no 'failure of imagination.'"

Jim's daughter, my niece Carrie, the Wyoming journalist, emailed me, "I'm rooting for a full recovery so I can read your entire comedic tale one day soon in print... you hit me in my soul."

My wayward brother Eric, who we'd dragged back from the edge of oblivion just a couple years ago, "Hang tough, love you brother."

Kathleen emailed, "Keep remembering there is more right with your body than wrong. I am lifting you up in my thoughts, expecting rapid recovery and a return to new trails in beautiful places."

John Reichle pointed out, "Nice to hear the crazy fun loving Jeff is thriving! You have an amazing wife!"

Text messages came from my brother John, Claire and John Zavgren. "Great news!"

Julie texted, "Awe, that makes me happy picturing you happy:)"

Lisa responded, "Wow, sweetie. Beautifully written and, I suspect, cathartic. Glad to hear that Lynn's over there with you breaking rules. Some things just never change. My love for you is one of them."

Years ago, before I had the capacity to understand what she was dealing with, Lisa's brother died from brain cancer. In another email she wrote, "He believed, rightfully, that at some point miracles happen. Often caused by science. It was a good way to look at his life. It helped him, and it helped all of us. It's how I continue, and how I look at your life now."

And from the chaos of their lives in Denver, John and Anne sent us a $500 cashiers check. It didn't correspond to any payment schedule or clear sentiment, but a welcome gesture nonetheless.

Then, finally, I had some clear cancer comedy success. My cousin Linda in California emailed, "You make me laugh. I'm raising a glass of Granach Blanc to you. Or, would you prefer a beer? Take care and don't run your wife ragged."

Of course, I pushed it and fell flat, " It is all relative, cousin..."

Jim resurrected the comedy. "The doc says you only had the mumps. My bad."

Not many days later, June 5, Jim and Kathi visited St. Louis, and it didn't take much cajoling for Kim and I to join them at "the cabin" belonging to Kathi's family, only about a 45-minute drive from our home, near Saint Clair, Missouri (not the new Saint Clare hospital). On a 75-degree sunny day, packing plenty of liquid food and pills, Kim and I wound down the gravel road to the cabin and the clear Meramec River flowing by.

In 1976, before Jim and Kathi moved west, I sat at an old table on the back porch of this cabin and wrote *Cynthia and the Blue Cat's Last Meow*, red ink on a yellow notepad, one scene enhanced in a later draft by a specific real life experience. Around 1983, Kim and I and Jim opened our eyes underwater, outstretched our arms and hands in front of us, and flew in the clear current down river, watching the logs, the fish, the amber stones on the bottom flying by. Left out of the story is the part where I took out my contact lenses, held them between my thumbs and forefingers, then crashed into a log and lost one of them. In the intervening years, Jim in Wyoming, me exploring mountains, the cabin was updated, improved and expanded. For a while the Meramec was more or less ruined by airboats and their wakes eroding the shoreline. However, recently, the river has made somewhat of a comeback, and that day in June, I may have been starting my own restoration.

Our older brother John met us there, and the three of us waded down river casting fly rods. We have done this many times over the years, sometimes joined by our younger brother Eric, and our Dad. And it felt good, even though my arms were weak, and I couldn't cast for too long. I caught a bass and waded back up river, through the grass, to the cabin, where we sat on the high bank.

Jim got out cane poles that he'd bought specifically for this moment. Seemed simple enough. Not too much effort. However, the bank was much too high and steep. We caught a few fish but mostly tangled our lines. We can cast a fly rod damn near anywhere, gushing cold streams, or slow warm water. You wouldn't think a cane pole would be so complicated. Kim sat on the bank in a lounge chair, sipped beer, read, and chuckled at our Three Stooges efforts. My pole busted, and we rigged our fly rods with worms and bobbers.

"Oh, the humanity," John said, heaving the bobber-weighted fly line into the current.

"What sacrilege," Jim said, swinging his fly line and bobber over the edge.

Kathi came walking across the green cool field from the cabin carrying a tray. Olive oil and garlic bread. Snow peas. Carrots. Dip.

I drank one beer, slowly, holding my breath. And I tried a small piece of the bread dipped in olive oil. I ate, tasted, and swallowed. What glory! Simple taste! I ate one piece after another celebrating each morsel. Even now as I write this I am envious of that moment as I struggle to taste much of anything, my taste obliterated by radiation.

I sat on the bank and said, "Get me the worms, I have cancer."

Jim laughed, but handed me the worms.

"Bait my hook," I said, "Because I had cancer." Then I started coughing. Jim and John watched. I looked at them. "Yeah, I'm always worried that my tongue will go flying out." My tongue often flapped, like a wet balloon when I sneezed or said the letter "L." Had my tongue become nothing more than dead flesh? "And," I said, "if I lean back too far, my head will fall off."

John said, "A Beetle Juice moment."

Jim added, "We can play soccer with your head."

Other than the cosmetic neck shave for the refinance, I hadn't shaved since April so I had a full, thick beard, and Jim remarked that I looked a little like Hemingway. (That image would change with radiation and he would then say I looked liked Bucouski.)

But we were having fun damn-it! Despite the three surgeries, my neck slashed open three times, and the specter of "horrible things." Just as we had in Columbia, Houston, and Philadelphia.

In preparation for radiation, on Monday, June 11, Kim and I went to see the swallow doctor. Professional, calm, businesslike Archie demonstrated my new swallowing exercises, twelve of them, ten times each three times a day. Near the end of the list, he showed me how to make the K and G sound forcefully.

I said, "Kim is Great!"

He laughed. I did it one more time before we left, and he laughed again. Hard to say what some people would find funny. Maybe he was just in a jolly mood because, after a year of being married, he was finally going on a honeymoon to London.

I did the swallowing exercises almost religiously, but they were difficult. See if you can stick your tongue out, keep it there, and swallow. Even if you have razor sharp wit, it's not easy. Try it. Often, while walking in public places, I would suddenly remember my tongue exercises. Probably I looked like the homeless schizophrenics who used to wander by Metropolitan School, tongue out, tongue in, Kah, Kah, Kah, Kah, and Gah, Gah, Gah, Ahaa EEEEEE!

On Tuesday, June 12, at 8:30 AM I got my superhero "radiation mask." Maybe because I'd been fishing at the cabin, and I had elicited a chuckle from Archie, this visit seemed innocuous. I was led to a room, took my shirt off, and was positioned on my back, all of it by now familiar, the only variance being the size of the machine. I'm not sure what they called this mask measuring machine. The others were CAT, PET, MRI. Just for continuity, they should change the MRI to a DOG machine.

I'm sure I tried a few jokes with the technicians, but can only remember them responding by drawing thick sky-blue lines on my chest, as if I were going to have open-heart surgery, and lines under each arm on ribs as if I had lung cancer.

"You do know," I said, "that it's my neck?"

They explained that the marks were to make sure my body was aligned properly for the radiation. Then they asked if I wanted tattoos.

"Really?" I asked. "Dragons? Snakes? Former girlfriends?"

"No, just tiny dots."

"What happens if I don't get the tattoos?"

"We'd have to bring you back here and realign you, possibly make a new mask, and put these stripes on again."

"Do any of you have tattoos?"

"Not me."

"Me neither."

"I'll take the tattoos," I said.

Other than my wrist tattoo pact with Andi, I had continuously vowed never to get a tattoo. But with a sound like a staple gun, pow, pow, and pow, I had three tiny dot tattoos. And I wasn't even drunk. Cool, huh. Now I could claim that I was stylish. I too, had tattoos. Tatooie! Nobody could see them without a magnifying glass, but they were there. I could prove it if I had to.

Then, without warning, they opened up what looked like an oversized oven at Subway Sandwiches, and pulled out something that had nothing to do with melted cheese. It looked like a fishing net. The technicians handled it as if tossing pizza dough, and suddenly a wet mesh covered my face. Then they whirred me into the big tube and kept me there for an inordinately long time. While I have never been water-boarded, I imagine this was what if felt like. But having naively gone into this mask-making venture, with no preconceived notions of torture, it was easy to imagine a spa.

After I was finished, I asked the technicians if people ever freaked out about the wet face mesh.

"Oh sure. All the time."

"Most people take something before hand."

Nice, I thought. I was exceptional. Didn't even need Xanax. Radiation was going to be a breeze.

Things seemed almost normal.

Jim and I were emailing about positive responses to his

novel. He admonished himself, "stupid to assume that NY agents grew on trees" and had turned down two legit agencies. We made the usual bad jokes. "I've quit many times" and "I'm perfectly sane." About his novel, I wrote, "It is very good literary writing and someone should want it."

On June 15, after one of our numerous doctor appointments, Kim and I met Julie and Daryl at Schlafly's Brewery, and Julie texted me later, "That was strong beer!"

I responded, "Enjoyed every swallow!"

I texted John Zavgren, "I have been eating and swallowing. Not using the tube. Doctor said I was healing well and to have a steak dinner. He said I would have to chew a lot."

Jim's wife Kathi emailed, "Do you know that I pray for you all the time?"

Even though I am not religious, I was accepting all prayers. "Please pray for me if you are so inclined."

I was overdoing it of course, biking, hiking, running. But my forays were short, albeit intense, followed by sitting, staring, napping. Almost no fly-fishing. Up to this point I preferred the sort of fishing we did at the cabin, sitting on my rear and not having to deal with anyone or anything. Going on a day long wading and fly fishing trip seemed too daunting. Protect the feeding tube hole from stream water, nap mid day, eat enough to avoid needing the tube, take my many medicines. It all reminded me that I was "damaged goods" and operating at only about 60%. But by June 22, I was ready to give it a try. I had taped plastic over my feeding tube, and rode to the Mineral Fork with my brother-in-law Brad, Beth's husband, where we met my brother John. Caught lots of big sunfish, a few Rock Bass, one smallmouth, fell in water, laughed about it, and continued wading before I finally told Brad that I'd "run out of gas."

On the drive back, I called Kim. Ken Yorgan had arrived from Racine, Wisconsin, in town for a chiropractic conference. Around 8 PM, I drove to Webster and met Ken, Kim, Lynn, and my son Sam for dinner. I drank a martini, a beer, shoveled food in, lots getting caught in my throat, but nothing too much to slow me down.

We embraced the spirit of Columbia, Houston, and Philadelphia, fun interrupted by terror. To those still working every day, it must have appeared as if Kim and I were on a perpetual vacation.

But radiation loomed. In a text message to John Zavgren, my trepidation was showing, "Facing radiation and not sleeping too good – a complex compilation of warring emotions." And by late June, the record-setting 2012 heat wave and drought was upon us.

On June 25, my brother John sent me a message, "Got kayak ready to go."

I responded, "Start radiation tomorrow."

"Good luck. This is the finish of the BS. Then all good. Receipt of this message redeemable for one kayak guided voyage."

On June 26, after a launch of a very different sort, I responded, "Freaked out but managed. Only 32 more."

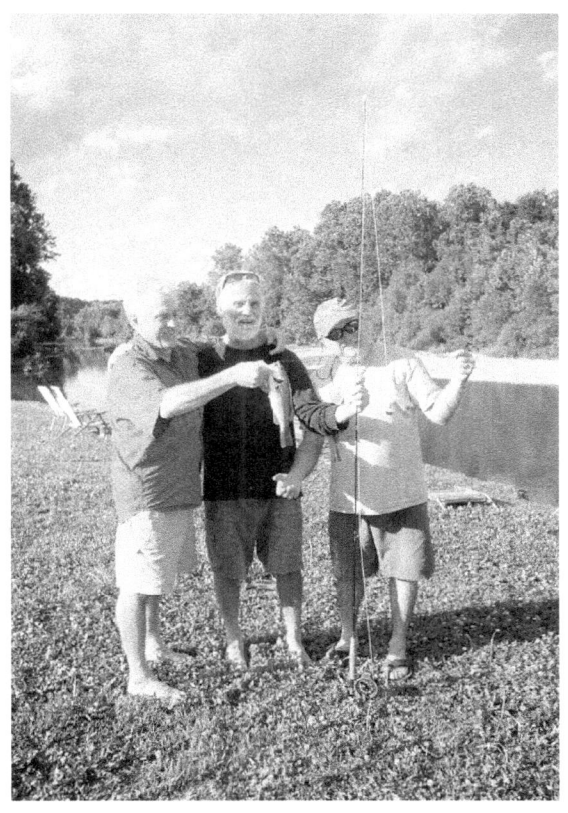

Jim, Jeff, John

Chapter Twenty-Two – Radiation

Radiation email June 27, 2012.

You guys would love this experience. I highly recommend that you see if you can find a radiation-ride-along program, something that allows you to have a wet mesh towel on your face for 20-minutes while lying on your back and tattoos punched into your chest, then two weeks later when the mask is rock hard, you can get strapped to the table and have the hard mesh mask locked down onto your face. And the ride-along turns into a radiation reality show.

The hard mask does not allow you to move your face. Breathing is interesting. Can't open mouth. Nose is clogged, dripping down into throat. This is the reality show test point. Who can do it the first time without freaking out? I eliminated myself from the show mere seconds after the mask was sealed down for a third attempt. They took another contestant while I composed myself. Composing myself meant taking the other half of the double strength Xanax, sitting in a small waiting cell, and listening to Kim tell me that I'd be okay and it was not a big deal.

Fortunately, these reality show producers are extremely efficient and the wait wasn't long. I went back into the big room, the radiation team I'd met the first time all smiling and congenial – they'd seen this before and they loved their jobs. I told the guy not to screw it up this time. They strapped me in, sealed down the mask, and hurried to their Houston like control room, the guy saying that they would try to make it quick, while I thought pleasant thoughts about fishing and having sex with almost every woman I've ever known... some of those thoughts more pleasant than others. (April? Did I know you well enough?) The Houston-we-have-a-radiation-problem reality show producers started their machines, and I could hear the whirring around me and my neck. It only took about three hours. Relatively speaking of course. When they were finished, the guy came back in, but didn't take the mask off until he tallied my score, touching my mask, his fingers like a spider crawling across the mesh looking for entry.

If you're only doing the ride along reality show, I'll bet you can opt out at this point. I, however, am in it for another 32 days, and I am soooo looking forward to my second mask experience today at 1 PM. In a movie, I'd be turning into a super hero. I think I'll ask about that today, see what they can do. What special power should I ask for?

John Zavgren replied, "Just like Alex in *A Clockwork Orange*. Next time, tell them, 'Give me that aversion therapy option along with the radiation. I want to be conditioned to have an aversion to Glen Beck.' (Maybe you already have that aversion.) But what would the 'inadvertent' coincidental conditioning factor be? Maybe the smell of latex gloves? Or the hum of florescent lights? Or the squeaking of a hand sanitizer dispenser? Or something that you actually love, like a well-turned metaphor? Or a participle that doesn't dangle?"

Ken Yorgan replied, "When I saw the title of your email 'First Radiation' I thought you had gone all evangelical on us and were about to expound on some new age church you had found. Thankfully, it's just a medical procedure."

Jim responded, "This sounds like a good time. Your Cancer Comedy has reached new heights of miserable happiness. The dripping down the throat part is called, I believe, water-boarding. I sensed your (acid) trip yesterday. It's that horrible depth of empathy that plagues me. I know it sounds like a broken record, but I believe it, and will say it again, you are going to be good as new. The special power you should request is to be turned into Miss America so you can fix all the problems in the world."

And of course I got other responses of support and love from family and friends, proving my repetitious cliché over and over again –again showing that what I often despised and railed against – redundancy – has turned out to be ultimate truth. On the other hand, I'm not sure love can be redundant in real life. Only in writing. "How Do I Love Thee" comes to mind. And the repetition of hate would be far worse, wouldn't it?

My second radiation proved much "easier" than the first. I took a full Xanax and lay on my slab while the machine whirred and the technicians stood and watched from their control room, and it was over quickly, relatively speaking of course. I loved the warm blanket.

Julie texted, "Thought about you today. Everything go okay at doctor? You drinking beer this weekend?"

And sadly, I had to respond I would not be drinking beer for "8 weeks." Drinking apparently isn't good for your throat during radiation. Once again, I thought of April, my accuser.

In the early morning of the third day, I hiked with Lisa and her two Irish setters. While we had obviously communicated, I hadn't seen Lisa in person for almost a year. True to form, she was running late because she "had to get some work out." Then, "Shit. Talking to client. Missed exit. Now in traffic. Laugh at me."

Lisa's life has always swirled around the excitement of the theater, her act sometimes blended with her heart, especially in those days that we were young, on the cutting edge of what we expected to be our stunningly creative lives. My friends and I came of age in the 60s and 70s, rushed forward with self-assurance and optimism in the 1980s, and by the 90s had settled into familiar patterns.

Lisa and I hiked, me with my shaggy grey beard but

healthy gait, and we talked, filling in the blanks of our lives.

By June 30, four days in, I was feeling good enough to talk about easy going things like the weather and catastrophic climate change, emailing Jim, "I'm fine but it's hellfire hot."

"Inhaling so much smoke," he responded, "in a sealed hot house that I'll probably never love a campfire again because the gates of hell have opened and the mountains are burning down; high 90s every day, week after week; haven't seen Casper Mountain for three days due to the smoke. So I'm doing wonderful too."

"Fires even here in lush Missouri. Doing well... but doctors say radiation is going to get 'tough' in a week or so. Nice to have something exciting to look forward to."

"You just have a bad attitude. When Job was going through about every ailment a human can have and then some more, plus the loss of all his property, death of children and other family, his three best friends showed up to console him but wound up telling him he just didn't have enough faith. That was his entire problem. Some friends."

The first week, June 26 through 29 went smoothly. No problem. I would breeze through this. They didn't know who they were dealing with. I'd been able to hike into the woods, and cheerfully drink my food. I mixed All Natural Naked Green Machine Juice with chocolate Ensure and gulped it down. I kept my feeding tube in because it seemed stupid to remove it, then have it put back in because of radiation. One week into radiation and I hadn't used it.

I avoided asking questions. I was successfully walking the fine line between knowing and not knowing, Kim as my pilot. I could maneuver my way through radiation by not thinking about it. That would fool everyone. Kim even said to me, confidently, "I think you are going to get through this without any problems."

Then on Sunday evening, July 1, something happened that I'm going to blame entirely on my cancer. Cancer has to be good for something. If it can't allow you occasional bad behavior, then what good is it?

I was trying to conduct my life as if nothing were amiss,

as if I could write, read, run, hike, and play like a normal person. So, understandably, I was still pushing it. Nothing new. But, because of the cancer and radiation, I was often exhausted.

I went upstairs, heading to my office so I could check email, facebook, twitter, news, sports, see how the Cardinals were doing without LaRussa and Pujols. Were they in a streak, or a slump? It was one or the other in 2012.

My son's room reeked, and I opened the door to find him and one of his friends partying.

"You need to do that," I said, "outside."

Sam looked at me. "Oh, okay, sorry."

"I just don't want you stinking up the house, making it smell like a frat house."

"Okay. Sorry."

I went downstairs, thinking I'd handled that well. I was clear and even and showed my displeasure adequately. I was an awesome parent. In the kitchen, I explained my displeasure to Kim.

"What happened to your sense of humor?" she asked.

And I launched into a self-pitying triad. "I'll tell you what happened to it. Look at me! My face is swollen, my tongue is numb, I can't chew, my neck is carved up like a Thanksgiving turkey, and they're stinking up the house" and so on, compassionately and affectionately ending with "So you can take your sense of humor and shove it up your ass!"

Kim stood and stared a me. She was smiling. Or was it smirking? She seemed calm. My wife is appallingly bad at conflict. And here she was smiling?

It seemed bizarre, until she told me what she'd heard, which was something like this: Ill at pap cook me numb tongue chew neck argh, ugh, mug, slug, cough. And more nonsense, angry tears, spittle and drool, arms gyrating, and the culminating "up your ass."

I stormed out into the nighttime 95-degree heat, the roads, the subdivision, the state, the entire Midwest, a fire hazard. We'd seen fires along the highway, and obese drivers flicking their cigarettes from car windows, reminding me of those wheelchair smoking patients with their IVs and their oxygen tanks. For the health of our patients and the public this is a smoke free hospital. Even at night it was hellfire hot. Radiation in the time of global climate change? No big deal because the radiation room was air-conditioned. What did it matter if my world ended. Everyone else was also doomed.

I apologized and blamed my outburst on my radiation and the apocalypse. The next day I bicycled, and my head felt like a bowling ball being stuck with voodoo needles. But at one in the afternoon, I would get to lie on my radiation table again and everything would be great.

Normally on July 4 we had neighbors for medium-sized, fountain fireworks. But this year, public displays were cancelled, and home fireworks would likely set the woods ablaze, flames to our rooftops.

Zavgren texted, "I hope the radiation therapy isn't too awful."

"So far, minimal side effects." Despite my discomfort, that was true enough.

Ken Yorgan wanted to know what I was up to and if I had read any Tom Robbins.

"Too hot for fireworks," I responded, "100-plus and dry for over a week. So far, no serious side effects. I've grown fond of my mask and am thinking about wearing it to parties. Working on my cancer comedy book a lot lately. I read *Even Cowgirls Get the Blues, Another Roadside Attraction, and Jitterbug Perfume*. My favorite character as I recall was Sissy Hankshaw with her big thumbs."

I texted Julie a happy birthday, "Hope you are having as much fun as you can stand."

"How are you feeling? Do you need anything?"

"I'll be fine:)"

By the end of the cancelled forth of July week, my stomach was cramping, sometimes severely. I asked the lone male technician about it.

"No," he said, "shouldn't be a side-affect because we aren't radiating anywhere near your stomach."

I asked Kim about it. "Is this what menstrual cramps are like?"

She didn't bother answering because she's used to my

ridiculous, sometimes stupid, rhetorical questions.

"Maybe," I hypothesized, "It has something to do with this constant 100-plus degree heat and our global warming future."

As if to answer, since no human would, in the early evening daylight of Saturday, July 7, I saw a huge bird expanding its wings into a smooth landing onto our street-side mailbox post. An owl.

I went outside into the heat, barefoot, scalding concrete driveway, and quickly skipped into the grass. I approached the owl. We stared at each other. I waved my arms, but the owl didn't move. I called upstairs for Sarah, our resident Harry Potter expert.

"Wow," she said, "cool!"

"Is it from Hogwarts?" I asked.

She laughed. "Maybe."

"So what's the owl's name?"

"Hedwig, but he was a white, snowy owl."

"Oh, this one looks like a Barn owl."

"Weird, he's just sitting there."

We watched for a while. "So," I asked, "what sort of magical powers do you think this one has?"

"Don't know."

"Do you think it can cure cancer?"

"Sure Dad, if you want it to."

I stepped closer, peering into the owl's expressionless eyes. It suddenly turned its swivel head. A car passed, the driver oblivious.

"Don't get too close," Sarah warned, "Owls are predators. He... or she... might rip your face off."

"You mean do a little more surgery?"

"Yeah, that's it."

We waited, another car passed.

"Do you think he's okay," Sarah asked. "I mean, I've never seen an owl land there before. Seems weird."

"Probably something to do with the heat. Lots of animals are wandering out of the woods."

Kim came out to look, and Sarah went back inside, getting ready to go somewhere. Sarah was always going somewhere. She was nineteen, and she had lots to do.

"Do you think he's alright," Kim asked.

"We can check on him in an hour or so. He should be gone by then."

But as the light faded and night descended, the owl remained. Sarah backed out, pulled next to it, rolled down the window and watched. Nothing. Four hours later, the owl looked like it had settled on its mailbox perch for the night. Sam had been out, and would likely be home soon. I texted, "Watch out for the owl on the mailbox."

"What?"

"Owl. Mailbox. Be careful."

Normally, I would have just let him walk past the mailbox and watched him jump out of his skin. But I worried this owl might attack, scratch his face like George Castanza's.

Sam was puzzled, as we had been, about the owl. Why would it choose to perch on our mailbox in daylight and remain there?

Finally, around 10 PM, the owl was gone. Just like that. What was he doing there? Did it have something to do with global warming? Or my radiation?

Maybe the owl caught a breeze on the mailbox. Maybe he was waiting for a Hogwarts letter. Maybe it was a sign, reaffirming my full recovery. Maybe, and most likely, it was nothing more than an odd anecdote to my Cancer Comedy.

The next day, Zavgren texted, "Staying cool?"

By Monday, July 9, I was feeling rough, my sinuses raw, head perpetually clogged, back of throat sore from dryness and drainage. It was all a big joke, exquisite misery. Hellfire heat and dryness and head ready to explode like a pinecone. But I was handling my radiation just fine. I didn't need Xanax anymore. The 15 minutes or so of lying on the metal slab and the machine whirring over me, mask tight on my face, wasn't as overwhelming as it had been. I was getting used to it. Sort of. Some days were almost pleasant, the warm blanket, the cool air-conditioning, meditating under the radiation machine. Other days I had cold press coffee jitters and post-nasal drip, but sinus problems didn't seem very gallant, often associated with sniveling, like the pseudo-religious guy in Jeremiah Johnson with his kerchief, wiping his nose on horseback while deliberating if the group should ride through the sacred Indian burial ground, all the rotting corpses on platforms above ground. Still, no need for Xanax.

By July 10, feeling microwave cool, I had settled into reading nonfiction books about deadly serious and often absurd quests, starting with *A Voyage for Madmen* by Peter Nichols. Even though I am not a sailor, nor do I have any desire to become one, this book gave me a sense of camaraderie, universal human drama, nine sailors in 1968, each alone, trying to circumnavigate the globe nonstop. The individual characters are as different as their boats, and only one is able to finish. If these guys could face madness and death, then so could I.

On Wednesday, July 11, my right side cheek was swollen. I had developed what felt like a dime size canker sore. I asked radiation assistant "go-to guy" Kevin about it, and he responded, "It's only going to get worse."

"Yeah," I said. When Kevin runs out of answers, he repeats himself. We discussed what could be done about it, and I swear, in the middle of his explanation about something called "Magic Mouthwash," he said, "It's only going to get worse."

And as he gave us a sample bottle of something called MuGuard, he told me it was "only going to get worse." And as we were walking to the pharmacy which is right around the corner from the radiation room and offices, he repeated it. I was keeping count. And I couldn't stop myself from saying, "Yes, I know. Worse. Got it."

By now, you might be sick of the "worse" line. One okay, two hmm, but three, not so good. More than three and it gets ugly. While I knew this instinctively, and avoided it, David Carkeet, author of *The Full Catastrophe* and other humorous fiction, clarified it and solidified it as a rule. He also told me that I often tried literary experiments, and I had to be careful of my experiments "blowing up in the lab."

So I'm blowing up that rule now and seeing if it works.

And soon, I was texting and emailing. "They were right by golly! It is getting worse. So turn that frown upside down."

John Zavgren pointed out that there might be some underlying purpose to my misery. He quoted his WWII vet father, now deceased, "Nobody's life is worthless, some provide bad examples."

And by July 12, I sent the following email. I hesitated in sending it because it really didn't seem too funny. In fact it sounded downright painful and I was leery about inflicting empathy pain on anyone.

> This one only going to a handful of people, about six, so aren't you lucky?
> Radiation side effects starting to have an impact. Hate to sound melodramatic, but... It is odd knowing that every time I grab the wrist straps, straighten my knees and hear the mental snapping of the technicians securing my mesh mask, and then the machine whirring and clicking around my head, that I am subjecting myself to more destruction, to expanding canker sores, and more concerns about post-radiation effects lingering, to pain and suffering seemingly without end – because 22 more days (and 8 "off" days) seems like an eternity. But of course I must go every day because in this quest for cancer comedy, I will one day find myself laughing madly, loud and vociferous laughter that will make me sound like a lunatic. Maybe I will have found myself, found the essence of who I am, the figurative gold of survival, the shining light before the end.

Lisa responded, "My sweet, sweet friend...my heart breaks to think of the pain you are experiencing. I am so grateful that your sense of humor wasn't radiated out."

Jim responded, "Anyone who says pain builds character or what doesn't kill you will make you stronger needs a punch in the mouth. Bullfuck."

Refreshing, I thought, to know that some clichés did not apply, specifically ones like "no pain, no gain." There was hope!

Jim continued in a second email, "Are you glowing yet? If yes then you are on the path to enlightenment. Your mix of comedy and the Spanish Inquisition make me laugh and cry at the same time. Is there any way you can forget about the number of days? To make it go faster? When I'm driving long distances, I avoid looking at the signs that say: 366 miles to Lincoln. It makes the trip and time go faster."

I responded, "Yeah, not thinking about the number of torture treatments is a good strategy. (Only 21 more!)"

From Lin Shook, "You know the deal. As an artist you have to constantly push to stay alive. Looking forward to playing with you all in August."

"I'll spare you," I said, "the gruesome details and concentrate on positive energy and remembrances of past good times, swimming though the silky waters of Michigan lakes, or the icy cold water of Lake Michigan, floating rapids on Missouri streams, all of the worthwhile good stuff. My last treatment is August 10. Hopefully, I will be sufficiently healed when you arrive."

Kim continued her constant research. MuGuard seemed to help, at least the online testimonies said so, and I thought so too but wasn't in a position to know anything for sure. Since it was new, and insurance wouldn't pay for it, she contacted the manufacturer and they sent six bottles for free, enough to last me through radiation. Kim also discovered that baking soda and sea salt rinses were helpful, and that cold press coffee contained the least amount of acid, and she researched honey, emailed a doctor in New Zealand who did a study on a certain type of honey, and surprisingly got a prompt response. (Was New Zealand full of smart, down-to-earth doctors like this one and Doctor Haughey?) The doctor said, unfortunately, she'd found no clinically statistical evidence that it helped.

So I used baking soda, sea salt, Magic Mouthwash, and MuGuard. I held the MuGuard in my mouth on the way to radiation, spitting it out while emerging from Kim's air-conditioned car into the blazing dry heat and strolling into the air-conditioned Cancer Radiation and Chemo Center at

West County Barnes Siteman.

Ten straight days of 100 degree plus heat! When I exercised, I breathed in foul air exacerbating the side effects. The St. Louis Post-Dispatch had front page stories about the worst drought ever and the record setting temperatures. "One barn in northern Missouri burned to the ground after hay inside got so hot that it spontaneously combusted." What sort of world would I inhabit when I made my full recovery? A world where we all sit inside watching reality shows, blasting our AC, while temperatures continue to soar, spewing forth carbon until suddenly the whole system shuts down and we clamor for "alternative" energy?

Screw it, I needed a haircut. So I went to the Hair Saloon where the stylist Jane knew how to be careful with beard trimming because she'd recovered from breast cancer and radiation. When she saw my scars, she said, "Boy, you're a mess."

I laughed and said, "Well thanks."

"You poor man," she said, snipping around my scars.

She was 72 but looked younger. Her cancer was in 1995 and she has been fine ever since. She also told me that a big patch of her skin peeled off. "They don't tell you things like that," she said.

I didn't ask her about other things.

Every Thursday, we met with Doctor Gay, and residents and interns, one with an intelligence, humor, and soft-spoken manner that bore an uncanny resemblance to our friend Barry Gold, a Barry-Gold-doppelganger. Likely, Barry won't know he's referenced here unless he reads this, or someone else tells him. I climbed three peaks in three days in Wyoming's Wind River Range, in 1986, with him and his brother, Lenny. Kim and I and the kids visited him in the early nineties, when he was in charge of water flow for the Grand Canyon. And not that long ago, he was in town with his daughter, visiting colleges, and I gave him input for a mission statement for the new underwater sanctuary off the coast of California, where he now lives, I think. I hope you will forgive the thinly veiled boasting, but I need to believe in the value of my life. That's what bragging is all about. We do it when we're feeling least worthy, don't we?

During these meetings, Kim always asked questions. I rarely did. Knowing how "worse" it was going to get didn't help. Kim asked what they thought caused my cancer. What causes mucoepidermoid carcinoma? She had asked this before. "Nobody knows for sure" was the standard answer.

This time, however, Doctor Gay offered a hypothesis. "They think it might be caused by radiation..."

"Radiation?" I interrupted. "So why are you radiating me now?"

He clarified. "Early exposure to radiation."

"So, what I'm getting now is absolutely necessary, right?"

"Yes, it's the only way we know to make sure it doesn't come back."

In another one of those "interesting" juxtapositions, Kim had been researching her Dad's skin cancer and eye problems, and found that he might qualify for a reimbursement of around 75,000 dollars because Richard "Dick" Einig was in the Army, assigned to the front line to "observe" over a dozen atomic blasts at close range. Dick and his men dug a trench, knelt down, then waited. He held his hand over his eyes and when the flash came, he could see his bones. The ground turned to a molten-like wave of dirt, overturning tanks, and burying them.

At home, Kim asked, looking up from her ever-present laptop, "Where did you live as a kid?"

Even though she knew me well enough to know, I rattled off, "Born in California, moved to Florida, then Germany and Austria, then back to New Mexico, then St. Louis."

"New Mexico?"

"Yes, Sandia Base. My Dad did some security work there, after he was a spy in Europe. They asked him if he wanted to watch one of the bombs go off, but he didn't want to go anywhere near it."

"It says here that you were downwind from atomic blasts, and that one was dropped 'accidentally'."

"I remember evacuating to the desert, but those were

drills I thought. Surely, it didn't go off?"

"No, I don't thinks so, but it is possible that you were exposed to radiation. How long did you live in Alburqueque?"

"I called it Apple Turkey."

"Yes, you told me that a hundred times, we've been married almost 25 years, remember?"

"Right. I don't know, I guess we were there about five years."

Kim made a file for her Dad and me, and downloaded applications for radiation exposure reimbursement. As of this writing, nothing has materialized from it and given the massive national debt, I doubt that the government is looking for ways to dole out taxpayer money. Still, if you like to look to the past for answers, it's an interesting theory. But right now, at this moment, I was more concerned about the present and the future. Full recovery!

Almost every Friday, the technician said something like, "Have a nice weekend."

And more than once, I responded, "I'd rather go straight through hell and get it over with."

On Saturday, my day "off," I walked two miles with Dave in the morning before the temperature rose past 90. Good-natured, occasionally dour, typically understated Englishman that he is, he asked how I was doing. Usually, during this process, I responded with a simple "fine." But for some reason this time, I apparently felt like giving him a description.

"Well," I said, "I have expanding sores and ulcerations in my mouth, my right side is swollen, my head feels like its clogged with mud, I'm constantly swallowing mucus that cramps my stomach, and I've four more weeks where it's only going to get worse."

"Good to hear you're doing well."

Near the end of the walk, my stomach problems returned. At home, I drank my Naked Green Monster juice and chocolate protein drink mixed together, then meditated for about 45 minutes, then slept on the swing outside despite the heat, tilting the awning to provide a modicum of shade.

Then next day, I woke with the side of my face swollen, head clogged, and I worried about the "worst." Worse than this? Holy shit! This was fucking bad. What the hell was I going to do when my face was swollen up like a baboon's back side and I couldn't do anything but delight in my pain?

On Monday, July 16, 2012, I woke at 4 AM, took Ambien, woke at 9:30 and went for a short subdivision walk with Kim, then went to my 1 PM radiation.

The technicians asked what kind of music I wanted and I said I didn't care. Then one of the women said, "I could sing."

I made a sour face and said, "No thanks."

They all thought that was hilarious. The laughter continued from all of them, so jolly on a Monday, as they snapped down my mask, the laughter then taking on a eerie horror film aura, the way laughter can when it goes on too long – Satan's minions.

Tuesday, July 17, I woke at 4 AM again, avoided taking pills, and woke at 9 AM. I felt terrible and took a very short subdivision walk. Then I sat outside, protected by the thin canopy of the porch swing, and read another survival story book, *The Lost City of Z* by David Grann, another confrontation with death and madness. It tells the story of Percy Harrison Fawcett, who marched off into the Amazon Jungle in 1924 searching for an ancient city. He was 57. (My age! I was 58.) He took his oldest son and son's best friend, and they were never seen again. Fawcett had already spent his life trudging through the Amazon, and had managed to reemerge from the darkness many times relatively unscathed, strong, ready to go again. What happened? Was it his age? Could I make it through my darkness at 58? Why not? Fawcett and his followers endured far worse than I would.

In an email exchange with my friend Robin Theiss, former President of the St. Louis Writers Guild, I wrote, "Books like *Voyage* and *Lost City* are inspirational for me at the moment. If these guys can sail around the world alone (many didn't make it), or hike through the Amazon while watching maggots crawl out of their arms, then I can wile away my hours reading about them in air-conditioning while the world outside burns and forget about my own skin frying and burning off and the gray whiskers of my beard falling out."

Robin owns an online bookstore, StLbooks. I write reviews for her Bookscape blog, and, invariably and suddenly, in books unrelated to cancer, the author always writes that so and so "died of cancer." It seems to occur often in narrative nonfiction denouements. These references never bothered me before! Now it's sort of like when you fall in love and the name of your lover suddenly appears everywhere, or when you lose your love and his or her face appears on strangers everywhere, or when you learn rock climbing and every wall and cliff becomes a route, or when you buy a new car and suddenly the roads are crammed with that make. Now, I couldn't and still can't bring myself to read cancer books, and cancer is in every book that I read. Doesn't that seem funny?

Probably because I took a Percoset an hour prior to treatment, I was jovial with technicians, comfortable lying down listening to the oldies station blast out early Beatles, "Yesterday" and then "Help." I listened to the machine whirring, clicking, and pulsing bursts at me. The skin on my neck was starting to look an elephant's hide or weathered leather. Only 18 more!

I tried to read *The Greatest Generation* because it was the generation of my Dad, and John Zavgren's Dad, and many others, but for me the writing seemed simplistic and the sketches repetitive, the same story over and over, as if repeating great great great. And I'd had enough of my own repetition. I got more from my Dad's writing, his account of Colonel William Cornog's demise, "The Death Of A Colonel, An Eye-Witness Account" by Walter W. May, 36th Infantry Regiment, 3AD.

By Thursday, July 19, I had crossed the radiation halfway point, and I was shedding my beard like a dried out Christmas tree, or barn hay. In the continuing drought and heat of 2012, I was likely to spontaneously combust. But the doctors said I was doing well. Sores in mouth were holding steady.

"My appetite isn't very good."

The Barry-Gold-Doppelganger said, "We can fix that."

He promptly wrote a prescription for an appetite stimulator.

Claire checked in, "Well, you're over halfway through. Hang in there."

I sent her a picture, my beard still somewhat in tact, but I knew that wouldn't last much longer. I asked, "Do I glow?"

"If I didn't know you better, I'd think I was gazing at a wise old sage."

Kathleen emailed, "Hope your are fast approaching the end of the red beam and dark room treatment."

But my beam was blue (or maybe greenish) and I'm still not sure if they change the color of the beam depending on the type of cancer, or the level of radiation, or the manufacturer of the machine, or another odd idiosyncrasy of the universe.

Jim and Kathi emailed, "We're still sending prayers, positive thought, optimism your way and we won't stop."

On Friday, July 20, my stomach hurt but the sores seemed less severe and we had a weather respite, a drop to the low 90s high 80s, and I went for a two mile Castlewood hike. I went again on Saturday.

Then I took an appetite pill, looking forward to eating. I felt buzzed and extremely hungry. I kept saying to Kim, "Let's go, I'm starving!"

We went to a Mexican place and sat outside in the relative comfort of the shade. We ordered fajita, with two powerfully spicy sauces, and drank watery margaritas.

The food arrived, looking good, basket of chips, taco sauce, steaming fajita platter, guacamole, rice and beans, the two unique and flavorful sauces in separate small bowls.

Kim dipped a chip in one of the sauces. "Wow, that's really spicy."

I rolled shrimp and steak into the fajita, dipped it in the sauce, took a big bite. I chewed methodically. With lots of difficulty. And waited for the sensual, sweet, bitter, spicy explosion of taste. Nothing. My appetite had been stimulated to taste dead leaves, dry dirt, and maybe, if I was lucky, mud.

I went back to drinking my chocolate Ensure and green goo mixture, adding various other juices, proteins, probiotics all mixed together in a thick liquid sliding past my wrecked taste buds. I sat in the heat, under the veneer of the swing canopy, and read *Unbroken: A World War II Story of Survival, Resilience, and Redemption* by Laura Hildebrand. Another death and madness story, fast-paced, a stunning and highly readable account of the torturous WWII events in the Pacific theater. The searing emotional and physical pain was rendered with all too much clarity. A harrowing read, and ultimately uplifting experience for me because – who was I to complain? I didn't even do chemo. What about those poor souls who succumbed to both radiation and chemotherapy? By Sunday, I had finished reading *Unbroken*, and went for two mile walk at Forest 44 conservation area despite the heat rising again.

On Monday, July 23, I woke remembering the poet Theodore Roethke. And I kept muttering, "I wake to sleep, and take my waking slow." I fell back asleep. "I feel my fate in what I cannot fear. / I learn by going where I have to go."

We went to see swallow doctor Archie. He gave me a plastic spoon and canned peaches, which I slurped down easily.

"How am I doing?" I asked, knowing of course that I was showing off for him, eating the peaches as if a starving castaway, ready to share food with a volleyball.

"You're doing great," he replied in his even calm tone, smart enough to avoid becoming too enthusiastic just in case a day came when I didn't do so great.

"What about his taste?" Kim asked.

I flinched, wanting to know, but not wanting to know, wobbling on my razor-thin tightrope, ready to fall into the abyss and flap my arms against the plummet, my only hope coming from an owl landing on our mailbox.

Archie said that my taste would "start to come back within two to six weeks and within six months would be 85%, but may not get any better than that."

"But," I said, "I'm going for 100%."

"Yes, some of my patients reported that. Some of it is

just a matter of perception."

"Okay then, I will fool myself into believing that I have taste."

Archie was kind enough to reveal a wry smile. Kim and I thanked him and shook hands and drove directly to my relaxing 1 PM radiation appointment.

Even though I wasn't using my feeding tube, I had to run water through it to keep it clean. I also had to use fluoride dental trays twice a day to keep my teeth from rotting out and becoming susceptible to cavities "for the rest of my life." I wore the trays and did my swallowing exercises while in the shower. And at night, I used Ambien. How was I going to get off all those pills?

On Tuesday, July 24, I woke at 7:30 AM, head clogged, legs hurting, struggled to get myself out for a short walk. I had no taste but the perpetual taste of salt. I had been losing weight, and forced myself to drink my creative liquid mixtures, and force down whatever else sounded remotely healthy. I didn't want to look like one of those holocaust survivors my Dad liberated. I swallowed my pills with my creative drink, Lexapro, selenium, B1, heartburn pill, stool softener that wasn't working. I then went to my recliner chair in my office to meditate, and I fell asleep. Two hours later I drank water and cold press coffee and then wrote for about an hour. My head felt swollen, sinus clogged and raw, neck fried, swallowing becoming problematic.

Fuck. I was getting tired of this nonsense. 14 more? Then weeks and weeks and months of more "recovery." Had 2012 become my own personal Mayan calendar apocalypse? Was this retribution for digging up those Pre-Columbian artifacts and smuggling them out of Mexico in 1980, just after Mark David Chapman shot John Lennon? Imagine. Have the savage gods come back to seek revenge? On a notepad, while lounging in the heat, I wrote, "Too tired and worn out to continue. God help me."

On Thursday, July 26, 2012, I sent the following "Radiation Update."

I know you all have your own hassles inherent in

merely living, especially in the current cauldron of suspicious weather (and suspicious alliteration), but I feel some obligation to email something if for no other reason than to satisfy potential curiosity. Mainly, this sucks and I really appreciate all your positive thoughts... thanks.

Thoughts with only 12 more radiations to go. Monday will start the countdown. After that, I will be in recovery mode, falling into the ocean in my mental capsule, slashing gently into the sea, hopefully near a vessel speeding to my rescue with the promise of good, quality beer as soon as I'm able to taste it.

More heat, and more heat, 100-plus degrees, while I lay on my back on the deck in the shade before the sun creeps into the sky and blazes down on my swollen radiated neck. Why not just lay in the sun on my deck, run an extension cord out to our old rusted microwave, disable the automatic shutoff, stick my head in it, and press fifteen minutes? We'd save gas driving to West County Barnes and laying under that expensive machine while I listen to an array of bad music, everything from modern country sap to Dean Martin's "That's Amore." Although, mostly I prefer Dean-O's amore – because the moon in the sky does look like a big pizza pie. Unfortunately, I cannot taste it. Nor will I be able to taste it for at least another month and then only gradually until I come to some sort of taste reconciliation whereby I have 85% taste function but have fooled myself into thinking I have taste. Not so much different than pre-radiation, is it? Still, I've read enough of neuroscience to know that even if my taste buds have been radiated right off my tongue, new neural pathways can form in my brain, and through habitually fooling myself my taste will return fully. (Although it doesn't account for my favorite piece of artwork being Seinfeld's "Kramer.")

But in a way, I suppose I'm fibbing a bit, because I do "taste" something and that is – Salt! I have a perpetual taste of salt permeating mostly on my right side where that huge tumor used to be. The key words being "used to be." Often, someone implies that I have cancer, but I'm quick to point out that I do not have cancer, that I used to have the big C, but I no longer have it because I went through hell to get rid of it and now I'm going through hell to make sure it never comes back. Through the skill of a great surgeon, I will be able to live my life "normally" much to the chagrin of the few receiving this email, or at least those who hoped for an improvement in my character.

Some have suggested that I "blog" this, and I've tried, but am finding that difficult. It's not in my nature to sprawl my little difficulties across the Internet, which would eventually mean Facebook. I get irritated with people who post about their sick cat or dog or their husband's goiter surgery or worse, photos of a colonoscopy. I don't mind anyone sharing my emails, but as I've mentioned before, my intention is to put it all together into a book, with the tentative title "Eight Billion Steps: My Quest for Cancer Comedy."

Robin Theiss responded, "You are effectively describing things in your weird quirky way with humor and odd imagery thrown in."

That was encouraging. Even though I wasn't laughing my way through radiation, it did seem as though I was on the right path. Perhaps my quest was not in vain?

Lin Shook emailed, "Which beer will you want to taste first? See you in August when things will be different one way or another."

I wonder what she meant by that? Never thought to ask her. Different? One way or another? Hmm.

Bob Johnson, an excellent Metropolitan School math

teacher who had recently figured out I was a mess, emailed, "Thanks for the laughs. I'll keep praying for you and your family, right after I remove my colonoscopy pictures from Facebook. :)"

So, okay, there was another bit of humor. But maybe it was inadvertent, I think I may have been serious about those pictures.

Jim emailed, "You S.O.B. I always suspected you were hogging some secret formula about writing."

That worked for me, except that I had no idea what the formula was. Was it near-death cancer suffering? If that's it, not sure it's worth it.

Julie's usual "fine" text message shifted to, "You're amazing Jeff:)"

These responses made me feel good. They were briefly intoxicating before reality set in, and then a tiny bit of guilt. (I went into writing this thinking I rarely felt guilty, but now I'm not so sure.) I couldn't help but think – so now I was like a rock star? Is that all it took to garner admiration, get carved on and radiated? Had I gained valuable insight? Understanding how singers, athletes, movie stars, and others get so caught up in their own false sense of importance, mistaking praise for entitlement, demanding adoration from everyone, including shoe shiners and spa attendants?

On the other hand, I have learned that it's important to accept the good will of others openly, without embarrassment, allowing yourself to return the feelings. If I've gained anything from this joyous ride through hell, it's that expressing gratitude and love can be liberating, and that while I still won't bandy it about carelessly, I will say it when it needs to be said, rather than standing around with a thumb up my nose.

I sent a photo of me looking miserable sitting on one of our plastic Adirondack deck chairs. "Don't I look cheery!"

Lisa responded, "You look sexy to me! I am proud of you."

My brother John replied, "You look good, like Pit and the Pendulum."

On Friday, July 27, my countdown began, 10, 9,

8...Houston? Do we have a problem? I was of course miserable, but "the end was near." And I was reading my next death and madness nonfiction, *Brutal Journey: The Epic Story of the First Crossing of North America* by Paul Schneider, Spanish "conquistadors" exploring from present day Florida to the Pacific coast between 1528 and 1536. Long lost tribes of "Indians" with wildly different and bizarre social customs, like science fiction. The transformation from prideful conquistadors to their naked struggle for survival and back to the "civilized" world provided insight into a time and place few had written about, and was another reminder of my own potentially dangerous quest.

On Saturday, July 28, I got up at 8AM and struggled to keep up with Dave Lancaster on our flat hike at shady Castlewood. I might as well have been wearing amour while plodding through a swamp. Who were Doctor Wilde's mythical athletes who trained for marathons while getting radiation and chemo treatment?

"Hey," I said, "Slow down a little, I'm having trouble with the pace."

"Really?" He was surprised.

"Yeah, I know, it's humiliating. Usually I'm racing along while you huff and blow."

"That's true. What's going on?"

"Maybe," I said, "It has something to do with getting microwaved every day."

My body moved only by sheer mental effort. I tried comparing it to nearing the summit, but this was different. There was no exhilaration inherent in the effort, no sense of being on top of the world. This was more like a death march.

When we got home, I took a two hour meditation nap in my office recliner. Then my brother John arrived, and he took me on a short driving tour, not more than five miles from home. We explored nearby Fenton lakes and Valley Park boat ramps, the river historically low.

Near the 141 bridge, we walked down to the water with my fly rod. I wanted to make at least one cast. It was noon, 100-plus degrees, full sunlight, no shade, mid-July heat and drought. But I wanted to cast, to try the impossible. At least go through the delicate motion unfurling the fly line into the hot air.... the improbability of catching fish as remote as my recovery. I changed my popper, tied on one of John's homemade sinking fly lures. But I wore out quickly, and handed the rod to him. He cast twice and hooked what we finally agreed was a hybrid white striper bass. He let me play the fish in for awhile. John said he should have let me bring it in all the way, but I joked that I was humiliated enough, having to bring in his fish. But I was inspired by the fish. When I say inspired, I don't mean that I felt anything at that moment other than exhaustion and pain, just that in retrospect, it seemed important. Better than nothing. A reminder that I had a great brother, John the oldest, the guy who had pulled me out of trouble when we were younger, and over the years. Although, as he pointed out, he got me into many of those jams.

On Sunday, July 29, while posting a review of *Brutal Journey*, I heard a gentle tapping against my office window. Rain! It was raining! We had way too many days of heat and drought. But the blazing sun returned in the afternoon, and I waited until 7 PM for a short subdivision walk.

Monday morning I celebrated, privately, my upcoming radiation number minus 10 and counting. Nine. Number nine. Number nine repeating like the bizarre pop songs of my youth. After radiation, I was wiped out and fell asleep on the swing outside because it was a "cooler" day, 90 and cloudy, and because I was exhausted from lying on my back and watching the greenish-blue line on the flying saucer like Zapper ease over my head through the mesh mask. I slept for about an hour, woke groggy, like I should get some exercise. After swishing salt and magic mouthwash and drinking my food, I rode my bike around the subdivision, then felt horrible. Weak. Body hurting everywhere. Pain pill doing nothing. Kim made me some chicken broth and noodles, celery and carrots, and that revived me enough to watch the Olympics and Jon Stewart. Then I popped an Ambien, waking to more liquid food and more pills.

Once, I drove by myself to Barnes West Siteman Center

Radiology for my "treatment." Usually, Kim drove, or Sam, or Sarah, always leaving at 12:30, up 141, right on Conway, left on Mason, right into the center, around back over the speed bump posted on big street signs as "Calming Bump." Never felt tense going over that bump. On July 31, Kim had to help her parents, and both Sam and Sarah had to work, and driving alone again wasn't appealing or particularly safe, so Claire took me to radiation. In text message exchanges, I said, "I'll try to be enthusiastic about getting to go again." On the drive, despite my swollen jaw and ulcerated mouth, I made jokes, socialized and felt encouraged. All I needed was interaction with friends and I'd be fine. Maybe I was doing this all wrong. Maybe I should have been throwing one party after another.

So closed July, eight to go. My favorite number.

Kim told me that we could stop treatments anytime.

I thought it an odd remark. "No," I said, "I'm going to finish."

She'd researched online that most head and neck radiation patients don't make it all the way through treatment. Another bit of info that she had mercifully withheld. But she'd had enough of seeing me suffer. She wanted to give me the option of opting out, of quitting, but that would be allowing the cancer to get off the mat and throw another punch.

"Fuck no," I said, "I've made it this far, I can go another week."

Doctor Gay and the Barry-Gold-Doppelganger were impressed with how I was doing. Maybe it was the MuGuard. Maybe it was the salt and baking soda and the Magic Mouthwash, maybe it was because I didn't know, until then, that most didn't make it all the way through.

I went into August with the idea I had only eight days of misery left and then I could begin my rapid recovery, running, hiking, and biking my way to happiness and peace, able to eat and drink and laugh and enjoy my enhanced bonds with old and new friends. Only eight more as in eight billion. Eight as in the dog ate my cat, eight as in, eight is not enough, eight as in infinity.

While hell fire was burning outside I sat in air-conditioning, running up a $300 electric bill and thinking radiation wasn't so bad. I had AC. At least I didn't have to suffer Japanese concentration camps, march through swamps and forests while mosquitoes and arrows pierced my neck, or suffer the loneliness of an around the world voyage. I didn't have to worry about an obsession, a lost city, gold, a prize, that inevitably leads to early death. Or do I? Do I still hold onto a dream that my fiction will reveal truth? What good were such aspirations when I woke daily, my head a bowling ball, my mouth a desert, and I became a leatherneck. But I was no marine, no conquistador, or sailor, or WWII hero. Just a writer with unpleasant metaphors. What has obsessed you? What dreams have you held?

Ken Yorgan emailed a suggestion that he and I and John Zavgren hike the Appalachian Trail in the Spring. The thought of doing anything other than sleeping seemed an enormous effort. I responded, "Maybe. I might have my sights on something more challenging, like a hike through the Amazon forest, summiting a Himalayan peak, or kayaking over a Brazilian waterfall." But Ken was and still is serious about the hike, as many others are about extending our lives into more vacation than work, fishing, cross-country drives, airplane rides to beaches, as if I was being paid for my illness and not the other way around, having lost wages, spending 12,000 dollars from savings, going into debt.

I think everyone was anxious for me to be finished. I knew I was being burdensome. Sometimes it's harder on those who aren't actually going through the torture. I know Kim had lots to deal with. But friends as well.

On August 2 Julie texted, "Is tomorrow the last? I've been doing a countdown."

I responded, "6 more. August 10 is last treatment day! Like your count better though:)" That smile, even on a text message, was an effort. And my treatment that day was prolonged as my pleasant technicians had to shift me around on the metal slab, even at this late date suddenly having difficulty aligning my tattoos to the machine. I swallowed mucus, reviving that wondrous water-boarding feeling, and I uncharacteristically kept my eyes open, watching the green blue lines of light and radiation.

On Friday, August 3, I woke confused, unable to understand why I slept so much and sought more sleep. "I wake to sleep and take my waking slow." Why were my neck and jaw swollen and why were my gums white and my skin like a rattler shedding? Why, I wanted to know. Why did the sun parch the earth every day and the water from the faucet flow warm from the cold? Why should I not run miles and miles in the 100-plus sunshine, why not run until I collapsed and melted away and flowed not to the sea but to the warm plumbing of my kitchen sink where I would reappear, where I would drink my own fluids, until one shining bright day during a cool off to 95-degrees, I become a normal age, a normal dying man, with plenty of life left in him?

Why were the hills burning and the crops withering? Why did the streams run low to a trickle? And the fish wash ashore belly up while the cattle collapsed, and we had to pay another dollar for our cheeseburgers? Why do we put cheese on everything? Breakfast cheese burrito, taco with cheese for lunch, and double cheese pizza for dinner? Let's go out for ice cream! Tomorrow let's get our fill of Chick-Fil-A, eat the waffle fries and fried chicken and watch our waists expand! Next week lets treat our Type II diabetes in the emergency room and watch our amputations! Why does the heat sear our folly into our brains while we pray for religious mercy but secretly hope for our man-made air-conditioning to cool us before the grid collapses? I was beat, feeling no joy in knowing that the next week was the last. Five more days.

Saturday and Sunday were a waste for me; they were nothing more than a waiting period. "Let's get on with it. Let's finish this nonsense."

"Have a nice weekend!" the technicians said.

The silence of the disarray around me in my office was deafening yet I could not move to organize it. Papers, books, supplies, wires, cords, glasses, medications all laying about me in chaos, no clean space to write poetry or poetic prose. No, just a blue screen where I posted absurd Facebook notices, occasionally suggesting someone buy one of my books, and avoiding any mention of Cancer, or my Cancer Comedy. My neck was fried, my tongue had sores, my gums were white, my cheek was swollen, inside stinging with lesions, and I needed to swish salt water constantly because "that's what I do now." Was this silly to worry about? After all, I was alive and the cancer was gone.

Would I exhale the smell of death for "the rest of my life?" Radiation does "funny things" to the bacteria in the mouth. What does that mean?

Claire texted, "Would you guys like to come over for dinner, and if so, what's a good type of dinner?"

"Thanks Claire, but unfortunately there is nothing that I could eat right now and even be able to fake it being a pleasurable experience:("

One of the few times I texted a frown but the frown came easily.

On Sunday, August 5, 2012, I drove myself over to Forest 44 and walked into the valley, then took the short route, through the green woods, hiking up the hill, slowly, and back, exhausted. I knelt again, and tried a simple prayer, but again I was terrible at it. Thank God prayer came from others.

I took pain pills. I sat on our futon in the front TV room, watching athletes. Am I an athlete? Skipping between channels, Olympians and baseball players, blanket over me, I watched their flaring nostrils and their muscles. I watched detached, full of inane thoughts. Why didn't that guy run faster? Misty May, why tattoos? Who designed that uniform? My thoughts matched the dumb-ass TV commentary. How was I going to achieve cancer comedy? What a joke.

Tears welled up, and streamed down my face, silent tears, impossible to control, the seeping out of pain that allows us to continue. Salty, the same salt from sweat after a good run. Same salt that was my only taste treat. One day, I will wake alive. One fine day I will see Gatsby's green light. And in that moment of eternal hope – Bang! You're dead?

My daughter came in and sat next to me, and rubbed my shoulders. "It's okay Daddy," she said.

Monday, Tuesday, Wednesday, Thursday, Friday. Five more treatment days.

On Monday, August 6, I woke in fear of what the week would bring. The weekend had increased my pain and overall sense of succumbing, but my tormenters would not get any secrets from me that day or that week. And Friday, they will give up, and I will ring the bell, and begin my long slow ride back to some sort of normalcy.

I talked briefly to Lynn on the phone and told her that I had a cascading list of ailments and complaints, so no use going over them all. Almost teared-up talking to her. Almost teared-up talking to my Dad.

Hemingway wrote a short story called "A Way You'll Never Be." While the writing is searing and poignant, and I admire his work, the title of that particular story always bothered me. It seemed presumptuous, almost like bragging (something he writes effectively about in another story where the main character counsels a young man). What I was going through was bad, but it's a way many of us have been and many have had it much worse, many cancer patients having to endure both radiation and chemotherapy. And what I was going through didn't match the suffering and courage of Louie Zamperini, or Cabesa de Vaca, Fawcett, Shackleton, Crowhurst, or my father. Or the slaughter, the starving children of the world. We all face challenges and this was just another of mine. Losing my first son 11 hours after his birth was a challenge. Being delusional and obsessed with becoming a successful fiction writer another. On the other hand, I've stood on top of 18,000 foot glaciated mountains, I've held onto my wife at 13,000 feet, I've known love, I have two wonderful children-adults. I have explored the highlands of Mexico searching for artifacts, and climbed in Alaska. I have lived a full life. I am grateful for the good times. And I believe, at 58, there are more to come. My Dad at 93 still makes jokes and smiles, and he's a WWII survivor, and my Mom survived four boys and being married to my Dad, and she can laugh at 92. So can the end be so bad? We always have a choice do we not? We can choose to jump early into oblivion, we can say we've had enough, willing to become the dust of the Great Plains or the swirling rocks around a distant planet. Or not.

I feared the next radiation because I had only five more. 5, 4, 3, 2, and one. Then I would be free, liberated from my tormentors, free to enjoy the exhilaration of surviving and make some sense of my life. That had always been and always will be a scary proposition.

Monday morning, my resolve faded after about a half hour of writing, after taking a walk down to the cul-de-sac and back and taking a shot of cold press coffee and pain pill. I struggled to continue. But after all, I was in the final stages of my treatment. I was at a low. When I emerged, I would be able to tell the story. I hoped.

Claire texted, "Only four to go! Hang in there."

"Thanks. This last week is really fun!"

And I clung to my countdown, Four, Three, Two, One and None. But I had no illusions that I would be just fine after the last day. I would have to recover from the cure.

On Tuesday, Sarah drove me to treatment and took pictures. I introduced her to the technician with the goatee.

"Can you see his horns?" I said.

The technician responded, "They only show up in photos." (I've seen the photos but haven't yet found the horns, only a slight cowlick.)

My brother John sent a text. "Short way to go!"

"Few miles straight up," I responded.

With just two more "treatments" remaining, I finally slipped off the sanity cliff, hanging on with my fingernails digging into the rock. I sent text messages clearly and eloquently stating my feelings.

"Ha ha ha ha ha! Two more! Ha ha."

It was August 8, and 8 is my favorite number because on its side it's infinite and it appears in the title of my Comedy, and there were only two more treatments to go.

"Go," I said. "Go."

Just after radiation number 31, in the car, while Kim was driving us home, I said, "Ah ha Ah ha ha ah ha ha aha ha ha!"

She gripped the steering wheel.

"Come on," I said, "Come on and get me! Bring it on!"

I might have freaked Kim out. She said, "You're scaring me."

"Laughing is better," I said, "than getting mad or crying."

"They all seem appropriate."

"Ha! Ha!" I said.

The red splotch on my neck had expanded past my collarbone, the sores, lacerations, and ulceration in my mouth expanded and felt as if someone were removing a nerve as you would the intestines of a shrimp.

But Ahhh Ha Ha! Bring on such exquisite misery!

It could always be worse. At least I wasn't dead.

The word mucoepidermoid kept popping into my head increasing in rate of repetition and intensity. As Shannon Nana the cancer therapist said, "The last week seemed to be the worst."

"That can't be her real name," Jim said, "Shannon Nana?"

> Sometimes I think that it can be worse for Kim or for you, if you're following this too closely. So if you want to trade places for a day or two, why not come to radiation Thursday and Friday? Maybe we can dress you up in my loose-fitting shorts, green T-shirt and silky bubbling beer shirt with the lime imprinted above the pocket. Maybe they won't know the difference, except that they have a lousy habit of always asking who I am and my birth date and where I'm being 'treated' to their sadistic treats. If you're interested, tell them that you are Jeff May, born 12-27-1953 and just wiggle your finger at the right side of your neck. That seems to do it and they allow access to the high-tech expensive machinery. Now, however, I'm back from radiation and will wait for tomorrow, and tomorrow, and then recall all our yesterdays and hopefully I will be enough of an idiot to tell the tale.

Jim's response was encouraging. "You're plenty enough idiot to tell the story and I'm looking forward to reading it."

By August 9, my mouth felt like I was sucking on razor blades, and when I woke at 3:30, I quickly went for the salt water baking soda combination which feels lovely at first, then the MuGard, then the Magic Mouthwash that numbs everything. I went back to sleep until around 5:30 when I got up with razor blade mouth once again, only this time I used the Magic Mouthwash, drank Ensure and probiotic and Green Machine, took a pain pill and Xanax, waking around 9 AM with razor blade mouth again. Pain everywhere, fighting panic, reminding myself about mind-body syndrome, how fear can exacerbate any slight pain and even in some cases cause physical muscle pain. I used the mouthwash and drank cold press coffee, flushed my feeding tube, and I wrote, "After today's treatment there will only be the last day, Friday, August 10, 2012."

In our usual Thursday doctors' meeting, they talked about how well I'd done and Kim talked about some-who-didn't-make-it, and then asked about the next steps. In a few weeks another appointment, then in a month, a CT-scan, then a month or two later, a PET scan. Those scans will scare the hell out of me.

Friday, I woke at four, then at six, then at 8:30, then walked. The temperature was cool, in the low 80s for the first time all summer. Then I sat in my recliner for an hour or so, fell asleep, disappointed that I had to wake. If we could sleep and dream our lives away, I would summit all the peaks in the world and feel the cool breeze of success in my face continually day after day until I dreamt no more.

After the last radiation, I thanked my technicians, shook hands with the goat-tee devil, and the others. They asked if I wanted to take my mask. "You're creative," the short one said, "You'll find something to do with it." Somehow, even though introduced at the beginning, my radiation technicians remained nameless. And even though they referred to each other by name, I never remembered them. I'm not sure why. They were all cheerful, kind, considerate, polite, warm, and my sardonic characterizations of them as "inquisitors, demons, sadists, and tormentors" never bothered them. They remained as warm and considerate as ever.

"Do you want to ring the bell?"

By this point I didn't give a rat's ass about the freaking bell. I said that my wife wanted me too. And, weirdly, as soon as I said that, I wanted to ring the bell as well. So they got Kim, and instead of following her out to the waiting room area, I followed her down the hall through a door and emerged into a small "crowd." Kim, Sarah, Beth, Brad, Dave Einig, and others were waiting with balloons, cheering. Balloons and posters. I was moved. Family and friends. What had I written about them?

At home, Dave Lancaster came over and was on the deck when I walked out holding the mask to my face. "I have to wear it for the next ten days, what do you think?"

Sam came in later that evening. I showed him the mask, and said, "I'm going to sneak in at night with this and wake you up."

"No, anything but that," he said, "It would scare the crap out of me."

"Yeah, I'd probably psychologically scar you for the rest of your life."

I got the following text messages:

From my sister-in-law Anne, "Bells are ringing all over Colorado for you today."

"Bells bells bells bells," I responded, "the ringing of the bells, ha ha ha ha ha!"

John Zavgren, "Still alive?"

"Let me check... I think so."

And others.

Claire: "Well, the fun is over. Now you can get on with the rest of your life."

Jim: "Hope you have fun tonight."

Julie: "How was your first day of freedom?"

Lisa: "Yea!! Treatments over. Much celebration ahead! Hallelujah. Feel joyous?"

Unfortunately, I wasn't feeling joyous, alive, free, or fun-loving. I was having a rough time as the radiation effects kept going. Maybe everyone thought I should be A-Okay now that I'd "made it" past the last radiation treatment. Maybe, I thought, freedom will come in slow fits and starts and that maybe in a week or two I will get a long awaited moment of exhilaration. Maybe.

On August 11, I woke at four, then at six, in pain, swallowed a pain pill, then took a short walk. I used MuGuard, magic mouthwash, and salt water. I sat in my chair and fell asleep waking at 9:30 when a salesman woke me. I drank my cold press coffee, messed around on Facebook, and tried to write cancer comedy. Ha. Ha.

That night was similar to the previous night, and I had a radiation recovery theme – I woke in pain at 3 AM and 4 AM with my teeth chattering. At six, I took a walk. And unfairly, ironically, I started using the feeding tube again. I'd made it all the way through radiation without using the tube, swallowing my liquids past swollen ulceration, dry mouth, constricted throat. Now I was on the tube again. At first, it felt like I was cheating somehow. Shouldn't I still be able to force my liquid past my misery? Just to say I'd done it all without the feeding tube? Fuck that, I logically and calmly determined. I'd kept the damn thing in for this moment, for this possibility. I just didn't think I would need it after August 10.

I wrote to myself – Now the tube that I wanted removed so badly a few weeks ago seems like a lifeline and I am grateful for it. Not that I can't swallow. I can if needed. But just the thought is painful. I don't want to try. So don't try to make me.

But there was something ironic and cruel about finishing the game, running hard like an Olympian, and busting across the line only to go on life support. Do I get a medal? Hardly seems to make much difference if you're dead.

I made it to the finish line without using the tube, I was still able to swallow, but the quarter size sore on my tongue was too painful to move, to flex without searing pain. I was spiraling downward the day after the race, and needed to go back to tube feeding.

What am I to make of my comedy quest so far? Am I near the end? It will never be completely over, because I will need precautionary tests, tests to determine if I should take a suicide pill because there is no way in hell I will do this again. Is that funny? Unlikely. More like a total and utter failure. That's redundant, I know, but so what, I've already admitted my guilt, that this is a repetitious, cliché ridden treatise.

How can I hold myself to my own impossible standards? I knew they were impossible when I started, but the effort might have been worth the effort. I still might find comedy. Perhaps on Daisy's green-lighted dock, or in some Shangri-La, on some summit yet to be climbed, where I can truly laugh in the wind at the continual joke of life and relish its humor.

On Sunday, August 12, in the evening, I went upstairs to my lukewarm shower for a quick hair wash, my neck burnt ochre, and my jaw started twitching, my back and chest hurt, my legs shook, and I struggled out, calling Kim, teeth chattering like someone dying on Everest, or K2, or anywhere in the Himalayan, the Karakorum range, places I dreamed of as a youth but only made it to 18,000 feet in the Northern Andes before succumbing to normal life.

Using the word "succumbing" is a bit of youthful bravado. As if the only reason I didn't trek off to the Himalayas and climb past 20,000 feet, and on further, into the "death zone" was because my lover, girlfriend, wife, was holding me back and then I had kids, and so on. But it was my choice, wasn't it?

And while reading Greg Child's *Mixed Emotions*, I had no desire to ever go there, and I was happy that I succumbed, that my family emerged to replace foolish aspirations. I am no stranger to climbing, and to dreaming, and reading about climbing dreams. I've read numerous mountaineering adventures, one that set me off on a string of mountain adventures of my own, Lawrence Lemer's story about Willi Unsoeld, his daughter dying on Nada Devi, the mountain that bore her name. I was captivated then. Now, I was crawling into bed, and my daughter rubbed my back and told me it would be okay. I promised my daughter that we would hike up a few Colorado "fourteeners," but no need to watch each other freeze to death on some faraway peak in thin air struggling with pulmonary and cerebral edema.

I wept, and told Kim and Sarah I was sorry. Apparently, I was prone to apologizing when injured, miserable, helpless, perhaps coming from when I was a kid often needing to be patched up, as I've written already, usually with costly stitches, my less than sympathetic mother worn ragged from my two older brothers. Therefore, I'm sure I got in the habit of apologizing when injured. It was my fault. And in most cases it was. Really. We should take responsibility for ending up on the side of a mountain freezing to death and risking the lives of rescuers and, if we die, it is our own damn fault for going there in the first place.

Monday, August 13, I sat outside on the swing in the heat in pain, watching my ensure mixture move through my tube again. I could swallow, yes, no problem, but geez, my mouth hurt, so why suffer the pain of putting food in my mouth. Salt on teeth like barnacles. I was gaining a new appreciation for the nurses and their exact measurements, because now my body was tricking me, and I didn't know if I was hungry or not. Maybe I would need to use the big suctioning hypo and measure backwash.

Of course I had been sticking my tongue out to inspect the "quarter-size" sore... and then became concerned about measurement. Maybe it was more of a nickel size, and I might be exaggerating, because our feelings sometimes distort reality and my pain was occasionally the size of a silver dollar, but if I wanted to be honest or at least accurate, it was only a quarter. So I decided to take a quarter to the mirror, hold it up and compare. Just to be safe, I also brought a nickel and a dime. I held up the quarter. No, the sore was definitely not that big. Not as big as a nickel either. Nor a dime; damn, it was smaller than a dime! But it had silver-dollar size pain. That much I am sure of.

Kim called Kevin to find out why I felt so horrible. Apparently, it was "normal" that the ulceration on my tongue was still expanding on the third day after the last radiation. Over the course of 33 treatments, radiation effects accumulate steadily, then the treatment ends, but the effects continue. The pain will "start" to ease only after I've reached the apex sometime within a week. I might feel a little better after two weeks. "Remember," he said, "when the first two weeks didn't seem so bad, well these two weeks after make up for that."

I was grateful not to have to drive to West County Barnes and be strapped down under the Machine with its alignment beams, its blue green whirring and clicking, although sometimes I admit to enjoying lying there and dosing off a bit, wasn't so bad. Other times of course, it was difficult to breathe and I had to meditate, redirecting myself back to my mantra continually. But this whole radiation thing was supposed to be over.

What cruel irony was this that the end wasn't the end, that the last day wasn't the last day, up to two-weeks of continuing radiation.

On Tuesday, August 14, I sent an email to a few, with the subject line, "When the end isn't the end."

I hesitate in sending you this email as I know that you think I'm "finished" with radiation and that I'm feeling better daily. If I were any kind of friend I would leave you with that image and tell you all about it later. No reason to inflict more complaining on you. But I am in desperate need of some hard core humor. That you are getting this email should be seen as a compliment of sorts. I need some wise cracks that will match the almost cruel irony that the last day isn't the last day. It's a false summit of enormous magnitude, one to two weeks of continuing or lingering radiation, wherein the side effects increase.

This was all confirmed yesterday when we called the radiologist's assistant, because I was getting worse instead of better, and he said that this period makes up for the ease of the first two weeks. So if you get inspired to caustic critical humor in the form of text messages or emails, I'm your outlet. You could risk a phone call but you might not be able to understand me or I might not answer. Although I am always happy to hear a real live voice. Ha. Ha. Ha.

My "getting worse" statement caused some confusion. I explained, "Getting worse as in the radiation side effects, not the cancer. The cancer is gone. The radiation is to make sure it doesn't come back. Think of it as a ski slope. The treatments ended last Friday, but the radiation goes on as I zoom higher and higher until I reach an apex, this week or next, then start to slowly descend to a safe landing (hopefully)."

Ken Yorgan provided the appropriate metaphor. "Kind of like when you take a roast out of the oven, it will actually continue to cook for awhile as it sits on the kitchen counter."

"That's it! The cooking roast. I was looking for a more apt metaphor as the ski jump one seemed just too cool."

Jim emailed, "You are in a war. You have won two major battles and you will win the others. Stonewall Jackson said something like: exhaustion makes cowards of us all. On that subject, did you know that the CSA Gen Nathan Bedford Forrest had 29 horses shot out from under him and survived the Civil War? You will survive, you will get through this, you will win. Right, most certainly, easier said than done; but you can and will do it and win. I love you, brother."

"Jim, Your pep talk nearly brought me to tears and helps quite a bit (that or I'm ready to go play football). So now Wednesday, August 15, the fifth day, I feel like I'm still cooking, or flying, but to fully mix the metaphoric pot, this might be the biggest hump day of my life, and by tomorrow, I might be ready for carving and beginning my descent into the after feast stew. Should be ready to cast some turkey scraps hopefully in a month. I love you too, brother."

Even though Julie is great at wisecracks, having at one point texting me a perfectly appropriate "ha ha haaa ha," I felt as if I'd leaned on her too much already, that she needed a break. I had explained to her early on in the process that I wanted to "spread the joy" around, not overburden my friends and family too much. So I avoided contacting her with the cooking turkey metaphor. But, rather than her usual text message, Wednesday afternoon she called me.

"Enjoying your recovery?" she asked cheerfully.

"Uh," I said, not-so-cheerfully back. "I guess I'll have to tell you." I explained the cooking, told her that I was hesitant to disrupt the fantasy that I was doing great. Then chuckled weakly, and said, "I'm sorry you called."

Then at 6 AM on Thursday, August 16, I caught a comedy quest break. I got up, dressed, and sat on the front stoop, hot even that early, and tied my shoes, noticing how comfortable and nice the cool morning felt on my thin legs. I looked forward to the walk down to the end of the street around the cul-de-sac and back. I stood, loved the overcast morning. We had suffered too much sun. I started walking, my short radiation walk, down the driveway and into the street, the smooth tight, yet flexible fit of my maroon running shorts. Maroon?

The neighbor across the street approached with her dog. Behind me, another dog walker.

I pivoted, and retreated back inside, upstairs, found my blue running shorts and returned to the sidewalk. Maybe, I thought, just maybe humor wasn't "impossible" if I had walked down the street, not in shorts, but in maroon underwear.

After my walk, I passed out in my recliner, and I dreamed that I was trying to fix a bicycle in front of Metropolitan School. Whose bicycle? Don't know. Dreams are dreams. The Director of the school was inside blowing gum bubbles and didn't know that I'd shown up for work. I finally made it inside, the bike still in pieces, and told her I'd been out there all morning. She had huge ugly sun burn marks on her neck, and she was chemotherapy bald. Of course it made some sense as she'd battled breast cancer in the mid-nineties.

My neck looked as if someone took a blowtorch to it.

By six PM Thursday, August 16, I felt as if I'd reached the apex, hit a plateau, stopped baking, and was maintaining a status quo, the exact moment as hard to define as the line between dreaming and waking. The side effects no longer, it seemed, getting worse.

In the morning, Friday, August 17, I woke at six, head clogged, bad sinus headache. I walked to my radiation cul-de-sac and back, assembled my feedbag, hooked it on the nail above the recliner, passed out, waking around nine, head still clogged, and feeling that this so-called plateau was just another false summit.

Maybe it was all the salt water and baking soda that made my tongue look like it was healing, but it really wasn't. And maybe that same salt-and-bake combination made my head clog. I felt discouraged and tried writing my way out of the mess. "I am so tired of being this way. I am going to say it. It. It. I am in pain, and I am discouraged, and I need to get out of myself, to do something that takes me away."

On Saturday, August 18, I woke at 11AM, and took a short hike at Castlewood with Sam, walking what we called "the bump" because it curved out like a bump following the river bend. We trudged through the deep sand to the river's edge. Sam started complaining about how difficult it was to walk in sand, and I agreed, both of us trudging along, then suddenly laughing about how ridiculous it was at that moment, the sand a great equalizer, both of us struggling to make our way in the sandy "wilderness."

We had hiked "the bump" at Castlewood many times, and now the bump on my neck was gone. There is absolutely no significance to that other than the semantic coincidence. Sometimes writers force meaning where there is none, and end up sounding foolish. But this whole endeavor is foolish. The moments laughing with my son, however, I'll keep those. Those are significant. I could be dead.

On Sunday, August 19, Claire found three versions of our marriage ceremony in going through files. "Want any?" she asked.

I was confused. "Versions of what?"

"Your wedding vows. I guess you took your choice."

"Who did I choose to marry?"

"It looks like you chose Kim."

"Nice to know I used to be smart."

I was experiencing a sort of radiation redux, or radiation rewind, many of the side effects going away as if in slow motion-picture reverse. My neck was molting, the sores, the swelling, the lethargy, receding imperceptibly. I wasn't supposed to allow sunlight on my burnt neck for more than 10-20 minutes, so Kim and Sarah modified a bandana, sewing elastic into it, and attaching it to my sunglasses.

Perhaps, I thought, I had a vision when I told Kim, "Bonanza!" This bandana was my Bonanza vision. Except that after they attached it to my sunglasses, I should have exclaimed, "Lawrence of Arabia."

I sucked a smoothie; it tasted like mud and sand. But I did successfully suck, a little. Still couldn't kiss very well. But I was okay with that because I only had to pucker up to doctors, nurses, and my wife. And friends and family, or anyone willing to do things for me.

I avoid phrases like "too be honest with you." It implies lying. When am I not honest? I can see the function of such a phrase as a warning that you're about to say something potentially offensive. I am writing as clearly and honestly as I know how. That's the whole point of writing narrative nonfiction. If I were to say "to be honest with you" it would only water it down and make it ineffective.

So... to be honest, when I was young and dumb around 1980, and striving to be successful as a fiction writer, a novelist, I admit to a vision of success that included beautiful young women by my side as I sat at a blackjack table in Las Vegas. Unfortunately, I was only a successful technical data engineer. Now it seems, success for women is measured by having studs at their side. It is no longer a gender question. It is what it has always been, a question of money. Money is success and success means money. Did I dream of that success? Yes.

I've always been competitive. And of course it infuriates me today when I see wasted words in "successful" money-making novels. Still, the only factor that counts in writing I suppose, is whether or not the reader wants to turn the page and is satisfied with what they find on the following page, all the way to the end where they feel sated and happy. The variables involved in that are infinite, and ideas for writing are equally infinite. They are also fleeting, usually arriving in the shower, in bed, on a hike, while meditating. In the rush to write them down, more often than not, they disappear. For example, I thought about radiation as a book review. But what would I gain? I'd already committed myself to comedy. Did I want to strap myself into a humorous radiation book review. Seems too convoluted to be worth the trouble. By this point in August, the enormity of my comedic ambition overcame me, and I wrote, "Cancer Comedy is difficult, but I feel like I must give it a go, give it a try." Feeling inferior to the task, I wasted about an hour reading online cancer jokes. A few made me smile, but I still had trouble reading anything about cancer and I couldn't find a joke that fit neatly into my narrative. For example, "Did you hear that they finally found a cure for cancer? It's called Death."

In another one, a doctor telling a wife that her husband has cancer describes how to take care of him. "There's a chance we can cure him with chemotherapy, but you will need to take care of him every day for the next year – cooking all the meals, cleaning up the vomit, changing the bed pan, driving him to the hospital for daily treatments, and so on." When the wife comes out to the waiting room, the husband asks her what the doctor said. The wife answers, "He said that you're going to die."

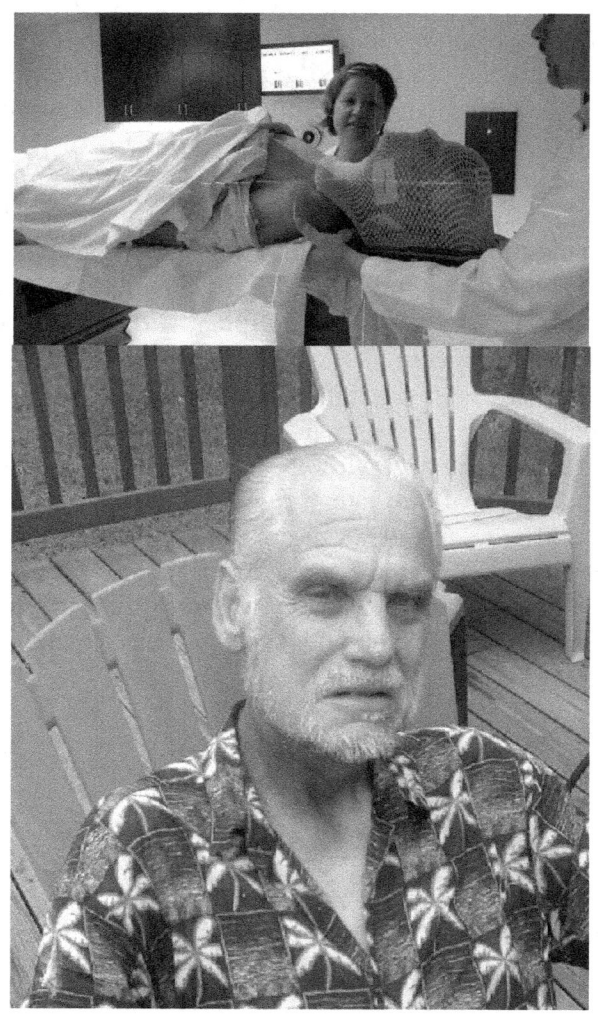

August 2012 – Ah ha ha ha ah ha ha ha ha!

Chapter Twenty-Three – Eternal Recovery

The right side of my face was thin and smooth while the left side sprouted gray. Shaving was one-sided, a lopsided game, an erratic appearance that matched my personality. Now that I was alive, I lamented the trivial, not being able to grow that thick Hemingway beard I had before radiation.

I woke at night with salty postage stamp mouth, drank water, nibbled on Xanax and Ambien, went back to sleep only to wake again, occasionally getting out of bed with a ferocious headache. Recovery was, and still is, frustratingly slow.

I slept late only to nap in the afternoon and watch TV in the evening. I needed a schedule, so I tried waking at the same hour every day, followed by a short subdivision walk, and coffee. (I no longer needed cold press coffee. That was progress, wasn't it?) Then I tried writing. I researched, skimming through reports about my big, scary malignant tumor, looking only for confirmation of what I thought I knew. I didn't dig too deeply because if I read the probabilities, I would spiral easily into panic, as if acknowledging the big C would make it reappear. What if it came back?

I wanted to live high on mountain tops where I belonged, forgetting malignant tumors.

Just a week after I'd hit my radiation plateau, Julie arrived with her positive energy and consistent support. She stuck her head in the door and asked Kim what the restrictions were. "Don't want him to relapse," she said.

Kim laughed. "Don't let him overdo it. He's been pretty good lately."

We hiked and shared laughs about our jobs, a welcome

respite from my daily recovery effort. In the afternoon, feeling somewhat normal from the exercise, I went to a movie with my son only to pass out later and wake with the same difficulties that I hoped would get better.

When Lin Shook came into town for her yearly three-day visit, on Friday, August 24, I welcomed the possibility of dependable fun. Dave Einig, Kim's high-intensity brother, was also in town, staying in our basement while planning his move back to St. Louis from Birmingham, Alabama. We were joined by Claire, Thomas and Lynn on the beach at Castlewood. Because of the drought, the Meramec River was so low that we could play in it safely. A few of us ate enhanced brownies, waded into the water and floated on tubes through the riffles in the sunlight. My Lawrence-of-Arabia scarf protected my scorched neck. We leaned back and let the current whisk us along to the edge of a steep drop off where we stood ankle deep feeling the current undercutting the sandy bottom. I knew the spot well. Many, even experienced swimmers, had drowned there. Each time, we could hear the thumping of helicopters, up and down river searching for bodies. I stood enthralled at the edge of this drowning pool.

The next day, when Lin and Claire wanted me to meet them for lunch, I responded, "Eating out for me is a miserable experience." They showed up later in the afternoon, and we sat on the deck. Because of my ulcerations, I had reverted to taking my beer though the feed bag and tube, the beer making me talkative, but the effects minimal because I was "out of it" most of the time anyway.

Lin was returning to Chicago and her dance company. When she left the house, standing in the driveway, I apologized for not being myself. She hugged me and said, "You are who you are, you're Jeff."

I tried keeping my schedule, walking in the morning, meditating, coffee and writing, but felt woefully unsuccessful. "I need to be productive," I wrote, "I need to be somebody."

Maybe, I thought, I could start by getting rid of my feed bags. I had only one left anyway, and our insurance was still balking at paying for them. So I went back to drinking my food, making sure I drank enough to at least maintain my weight. I'd lost about 35 pounds since January 2012. And of course, at every opportunity, I recommended my diet plan. "Side effects are tough, but you will lose weight. It's a wonderful diet."

And, regardless of my "situation," daily life-concerns of course continued, including problems with aging parents. On my Mom's birthday, the same date as my brother John's, she was taken away, unwillingly, by ambulance, her behavior erratic and uncharacteristic, refusing to go to the neurologist, the signs of dementia. Because sustained effort on anything was extremely difficult for me, I could only offer support by phone and email.

My parents were a concern, and so were my children, Sam still not sure about his future, and Sarah ready to jump into life full force (with her boyfriend). She and Kim were working hard on finding an apartment in Denver, while I went to the next doctor appointment on my own.

I asked about my inability to taste.

"Try a beer you don't like," Kevin suggested.

"That might be difficult," I responded.

"It might work," the doppelganger said, "A bitter taste, one that your taste buds are sensitive to."

"Yeah," I said, "But as far as I know, there aren't any beers I don't like." Which was a lie, of course. My Dad and I were on a back gravel road deep in the Ozarks going from stream to stream and meeting up with my brothers when we decided to "taste" Bud Lite following a beer connoisseur's guidelines. We promptly poured it out onto the gravel and bought some "real" beer.

"I want," I said, "my tube out."

"Who put it in?" Doctor Gay asked.

"I've had it in since April, so... Doctor Haughey."

"Usually, we don't take out a tube someone else put in."

"Oh come on," I said, "You can do it." I pulled up my shirt. "Here. You guys grab hold and yank."

Even though they were reluctant, they scheduled a tube removal. I celebrated by doing what I would have done anyway, hiking, interspersed with running, then I waded the super low Meramec, and caught one smallmouth. Dave Lancaster and Kathleen Hudson arrived on the deck, and I ignored the feeling of being constantly strangled, drank a beer through my mouth and almost felt good, the stinging not as bad as it could have been. Suddenly, I could taste the India Pale Ale. And I loved IPA! I considered fulfilling April's dream and getting drunk and staying drunk for a long time. And so ended August – radiation completed, intense side effect receding, shifting to the long slow process of full recovery.

Early in September, Kim and Sarah drove to Denver to look for apartments, Dave Einig went back to Alabama for a few days, and Sam was working. So I called to see if I could drive myself to my tube removal.

"Yeah," Kevin said, "Maybe."

"So I can drive okay."

"Yeah, but just to be safe, I'd have someone drive you."

"Okay..."

"Just in case."

"Of what?"

"You never know about these things."

So Julie drove me to West County Barnes for my feeding tube removal, and waited until they took me away, ha ha. I'd call or text when finished.

A nurse took me to what looked like partitioned office cubical along a hallway and about the size of a closet. She sat me in a metal chair suitable for auditoriums, and told me to pull up my shirt.

"Oh," she said, looking at the tube, "I think we can do that here."

"Okay," I said, glancing around, people skirting past the cubicle. "Sure, why not."

An intern arrived immediately. "Is there a balloon?" he asked.

"A balloon?"

"Some have balloons on the inside to hold the tube in place."

"I had stitches," I said, thinking about big balloons in

my stomach, and floating away into the clouds. "But they're gone now... came out when I stepped on my tube."

"This should be easy then."

He turned away, opened a drawer in a movable tool cart, and then he came at me with a pair of scissors. They looked like ordinary kitchen scissors. He snipped off the end of the tube. I braced myself as he grabbed the tube and yanked it out, apparently with a just-so turning motion. That was it. No anesthesia, no pain pills, nothing. My "yanking" suggestion to Doctor Gay and the others turned out to be true. They could have done it a week ago. I could have done it myself in the shower. Provided of course I knew the right turning motion. The end of the tube looked like a boat-dock post pulled from the water, smelled like one too. They taped a piece of gauze over the hole, but said it would close up almost immediately. "Will beer squirt out?" I asked.

The "procedure" took about five minutes. I was hurrying along the hallway and dialing Julie who had just driven out of the parking lot, now making a U-turn. I skipped energetically out to the car and climbed in.

"That's it?" she asked.

"Yeah, sort of anti-climatic, isn't it? Sorry. I could have driven myself."

"Yeah, I wanted to feel like I was at least needed. Could you limp or something?"

I was free from the tube, another stride toward some semblance of normalcy, the "hole" closing up like they said – immediately. That didn't stop me from joking about being a cartoon character shot full of holes and liquid squirting out.

One morning, we had a misty rain, not much but more that it had rained all summer, and I started thinking about the looming follow-up scans. Even though the first scan was more than a month away, I was suddenly consumed with doubt. What if the C cells had hidden in my nerves?

At my last appointment, I'd asked the Barry-Gold-doppelganger, "It's just standard operating procedure, right?"

"Ah, yeah, but it needs to be done."

If I thought about it too much, I realized his answer was

hardly definitive. I wanted to hear him say, "Yes, SOP, no way it will show anything."

Later, while walking in the mist, I muttered, "Please dear God, don't put my wife through this again."

No doubt my wife deserved some respite, but there was nothing noble, nothing selfless in my prayer. Not at all. It was just easier to pray for others. Not that I didn't try praying for myself. I'm just not very good at it. Praying for myself would force me to find worth in my life, to ask difficult questions. Why did I deserve to live when so many others suffered and died?

I often laid in bed thinking about myself and God. I took long showers and talked to myself, out loud sometimes, and I wondered if I was I speaking to God. I thanked God every day for my wife, my kids, my brothers, Mom and Dad, friends, grocery store clerks and even politicians. Alone, under the noise of the shower's hot water on my head, I said, "Thank you God." Once I tried a Christian slant. "Thank you my lord and savior Jesus Christ."

But this was unfamiliar territory for me and, while necessary, did not appear in any "clinical study." My beliefs still hinged on something more nebulous than a person. If anything, I believed in science, technology, secular morality, nature and neurobiology, everything in the universe. My body, my brain, will one day stop and deteriorate like a discarded car or computer, all mass continuing to exist, just in a different form. But will I lose my mind? Will my synapses flash and disappear "across the universe?" Nothing's gonna change my world.

Logically, I understand, even embraced, how belief can affect reality. After all, I asked everyone to believe in me. I welcomed their prayers, encouraged them to pray. People who knew me only as a concept, someone's son, brother, friend, prayed for me. And I am forever grateful. Prayer meant belief, and I desperately needed to believe in my full recovery.

Sure, I was forced to my knees, and I felt like quitting. Would that be giving in to God, or merely be giving up, the act of quitting reinterpreted as "God's will?" The surgeons, nurses and technicians, did not (I hope) throw up their hands and say, "Jesus take the wheel." Was my survival the work of God, or was it Doctor Haughey's dedication and skill, his constant striving to be the best, his humility? What sort of human being would I be if I did not thank the surgeon, the horned technicians, even April who failed but who deserves to be acknowledged for her attempt, her avocation? And what role did God's hand take in the development of anesthetic, lasers, TORS, advanced medicine superseding whiskey and dirty knives?

Thank God... we have ever evolving neurobiology allowing us to believe in ourselves and to work hard for a better world. So I hiked and ran and cussed, and worked hard on my recovery because I believed.

At our first meeting after radiation, I looked at Doctor Haughey and said, "That was fun."

He smiled.

Then I said, "I don't want to do that again."

"Lucky for you," he replied, "it's a one-time thing."

He looked in my mouth, gathered his interns and residents, and using my tongue as a teachable moment, pointed out how everything looked good.

"How are you coming along?" he asked.

"I did run two miles, but still don't feel right."

"Right," he said, "Most people would be very happy running two miles a few weeks removed from radiation."

We joked about the next appointment in four months, how I was relieved because I wouldn't have to see him for a long time. I was afraid to ask about the upcoming scans.

Finally, my brother John and I took his kayak on the Meramec from Sherman Beach to Castlewood. The river suddenly swollen after 6.5 inches of recent rain from hurricane Isaac, its highest mark all summer, enough to make the river briefly flow fast and deep. I believed there were fish to be caught and I cast my fly rod. From the muddy bottom, I caught a large mussel.

On Sunday morning, September 23, I was putting in my contact lenses when I noticed that my neck on the left side was swollen. I freaked. "It's coming back," I said. Kim reassured me it wasn't. I went for a subdivision walk. Every half hour, I asked her if it was still swollen. I asked my basement brother-in-law Dave Einig.

"You can drive yourself crazy with that sort of stuff," he said.

"I know, I'm good at driving myself crazy."

What if a tumor was growing on the left side? What if I had to go through more surgery? Kim quickly researched it and found that I had lymphedema, common when lymph nodes have been removed or subject to radiation. I should avoid long hot showers (with God?)

By October, my psyche was erratic as I struggled through this extremely frustrating phase of my recovery. Irritating side effects lingering on for an eternity. I was tortured by a thousand cuts, headaches, neck zinging stinging burning pain, tongue rough and swollen, jaw swollen, little taste, and so on, frustrated waking up every day with sinus headaches and now lymphedema. Yeah, okay, a side effect, but damn-it, enough of those.

My younger brother Eric let us borrow his truck so we could move my daughter and her boyfriend Dominic to Denver. Before their departure, they hiked with me along the bluffs overlooking the Meramec snaking in from the west, and we discussed their move. Although no one is ever good enough for my little girl, I was encouraged by their pragmatism and optimism. I told them that regardless of where they were in ten years, this was good for them. So, looking like the Beverly Hillbillies, Kim and I drove the truck, followed by Sarah in her car, Dominic in his, straight through to Denver, to Anne and John's, where we revived a smattering of the good old times before the Great Recession and Cancer.

My daughter's apartment is on Poet's Row in downtown Denver. I told Sarah that I envied her. I'd love to be 20 and moving to Denver. I told her I was happy she was following her dream. She worked at Starbucks, will go to community college after she establishes residency, then possibly to Denver University or Boulder if we can find the money.

On our last day in Denver, Sarah drove me to Rocky

Mountain National Park, up along the Trail Ridge Road. We stopped and watched about ten big horn rams wander close by, and we hiked a short trail in the strong freezing wind, up to about 12,000 feet, my daughter and I. We watched hundreds of elk wander through meadows, bleating, unwieldy multi-pointed racks, calf suckling. On the drive back, I had the eerie feeling that it could be the last time she and I would be in the mountains together. What value should we put into such premonitions? I fought it, vowing that this summer, 2013, we would climb a "fourteener." I told her I would miss her and love her always, and that she would always be my little girl. I am so proud of her. This was "normal." This was my life. I was getting there, wasn't I?

But I still didn't have the endurance for long-distance driving, and Kim had to navigate through Kansas City at night. A day after the grueling drive home, Kim flew to Birmingham to help her brother move, figuring it would help her forget the hole in her heart from Sarah's departure.

The last radiation was more than two months ago. Two months and 12 days. So why wasn't I back to 100%? Would I be able to work in January? Sometimes when I ate, my tongue hurt, and a zombie still had its hands perpetually around my neck.

On Monday, October 22, I got up at six, went for a walk, came back and fell asleep until 10, then went in for the CAT scan.

I reverted to the sort of humor one has prior to the hellish trip I'd been on, as if I were merely donating blood. To the nurse, Michelle, stabbing me with the IV, I said, "So you've done this before?"

And she laughed! "Yeah," she said, "I saw the video."

"I'll bet you've heard that joke before too." Then I explained my surgery, why I was getting the scan, and how I slept poorly the past couple nights. "I was terrified," I said, "because I heard stories about a nurse named Michelle. You're all over the Internet."

She laughed, and I was feeling downright normal. There was a chain across the door to a scan in progress. "Is that the same chain you use on your patients?"

Michelle said, "You're funny."

And I thought, yes, about as funny as anybody could be facing the possibility of another trip to hell. Funny in a funny sort of way. My father told me about a time when he was called to a meeting on the battlefield, officers standing around in the open, "crazy," my Dad said. And a shell hit nearby. "Gee," my Dad said, "if I didn't know any better, I'd think they were shooting at us." The Colonel stared grim-faced and did not see the humor. Shortly after, a shell hit their group, and the Colonel was fatally wounded, lying on the battlefield begging my father, "Don't leave me." Funny how those things work out.

After the scan, I asked the technician when the results would be ready.

"Today," she said, "But we need to send them to your doctor, so maybe tomorrow."

And I thought... *tomorrow creeps in this petty pace from day to day... a tale told by an idiot, full of sound and fury, signifying nothing.*

On the morning of Tuesday, October 23, I should have called for results. Instead, I escaped into this comedy, because it was all so hilarious. I needed to gather the courage to call. I could go on the assumption that as long as I didn't know anything, everything was okay. But that method didn't work so well with my son in January when he forced me to face the truth. Would I now be fulfilling my prognostication? "I'm going to suffer a slow and painful death."

There was no reason to think the scan would show anything untoward. But if there was no reason to think that, why do the scan in the first place? What's the point? What could be done if it shows something? Hmm? What then? Doctor Haughey said no more radiation, that radiation was a "one time shot." So why bother?

So, instead of calling for "results," I wrote, and prepared for my return to work. We were burning through our savings. If we had not worked our entire lives, made the right moves, and understood the importance of health insurance, I'd be severely maimed or dead. In cynical moments, I'd think that everything was all about the money. A big change from what

I told Kim in 1987 when we quit our jobs to become teachers. "It's easy to make money, it's about how you make the money." But now of course I have experience, and age. Money buys health care. Money can't buy you love, but it sure helps. No big revelation there.

I focused on my parents, trying to get them help, and that focus spiraled into a vision of Kim and I, old like our parents. I imagined that we might traipse into the wilderness and fall to our knees before a crashing waterfall. We will all give in eventually, and very likely I will pray to God for eternal salvation.

After the big operation, the doctors told Kim that when cancer gets in a nerve like mine had, the odds diminished, but warned her not to look at it that way. People who didn't take care of themselves skewed the statistics. Obviously, they said, I was in great shape. Kim added, that even if it did come back, likely it would be too small to show up on a scan, and that she would be more worried about tests three years from now. What the hell was she doing? Maybe she couldn't hold back "info" anymore. Had I asked too much of her?

At noon, Kim called Kevin, got voicemail, and left a message that she would call back at 2:30. I decided to ride my bike down the hill to look at the new bridge construction over Fishpot Creek, muddy backhoe and bulldozer. I was feeling pretty good, so I went for a longer ride. At 2:37, I called Kim and got no answer. Shit! What if the news was bad and she wasn't answering her phone until I came home so she could tell me face to face? What if she thought that if she told me on the phone I might commit suicide by riding my bike into the teeth of the construction-site bulldozer?

In a full-blown panic, I peddled up the hill and home and rushed inside, "Kim!" I shouted. Nothing. I went upstairs. She was on the phone. I waited. She must, I thought, be listening to the gruesome test results. After excruciating minutes, I realized that she was talking to her sister Beth; they were involved in one of their long conversations.

I went back out and rode around the subdivision,

avoiding the hill this time, talked to a neighbor, and came back. She was still on the phone. I went outside onto the deck, stood, went into my office, checked email, then started vacuuming. I was scared. Back to the bike, then inside at 3:30.

Kim had called and left another voice message. She also called Doctor Haughey's assistant and left a message. At 4 PM, I couldn't stand it any longer and knew that if I didn't find out, I'd be up all night. I called, and Kevin answered in his always kind and cheerful manner.

"Oh," he said, "I haven't had a chance to check on those."

He put me on hold. I waited as long as I could stand, then handed the phone over to Kim. I paced our daughter's empty room.

Then I heard Kevin's loud friendly voice.

All clear. No Cancer!

I smacked my hands together. I whooped. Hollered. Shed tears.

"We beat it," I said, "didn't we?"

"Yes," Kim said. "We did."

We hugged. Aside from the left-side test trial, which seemed long ago, this was the first time we'd had a test showing I was cancer-free.

On Wednesday, October 24, Lynn, Lisa, her husband Shane, Claire, and Thomas came over to celebrate our 25th anniversary. Except Thomas, they'd been at our wedding in 1987. While I wasn't as interactive as I might have been, somehow life was good. I loved my wife more than I ever have.

In an email exchange with my brother Jim, we talked about baseball. I had moved on to reading *Three Nights in August*, baseball a little less harrowing than stories of survival. The Cardinals had lost to World Series winner San Francisco, and I wrote, "Relieved when the Cardinals peculiar brand of baseball was over because it indicated to me that my travels into the bizzaro world might be over as well."

On Thursday, November 1, I went to the Lymphedemia

physical therapist, Shelly Ryan, the start of two and three times a week through the holiday season when she pulled, pushed and twisted my scars and my lymph nodes to the tune of "We wish you a Merry Christmas." She gave me homework for my mouth and jaw: stretch neck, wear her customized "strap" six hours preferably while sleeping (looked a lot like my old bandages), yawn a lot, chew more gum (which further blunted my taste), shove eight tongue depressors between molars until you could fit about twenty. I enjoyed visiting her, even dozing off while she pulled and twisted, comfortable enough to float a musing question about my facial hair, since I noticed some was growing back. She said that I might grow hair. Said that only about 20% don't get it back. Nice, I thought, I might be able to grow that thick beard, if I wanted.

I also visited Shannon Nana. She talked about out how well I was doing, however, I set my expectations impossibly high. She was right of course. No surprise there. But therapy is often all about allowing yourself to accept the obvious, and adjusting your perspective. Shannon Nana was helpful. But she was moving to the Antilles, taking a professorship there. We scheduled one more visit just before my numerological nemesis, November 22nd.

Were "things" getting better? Yes, they were. I wrote for about two and a half hours in the morning. I worked in the basement. I cleaned the bathroom. I ran two miles fast. I went to the grocery store, came home and made chili. I watched "The Walking Dead" and football. I sent emails, played politics on FB, and even though we could ill afford it, planned a trip to Hot Springs, Arkansas.

After voting, we drove to Hot Springs, and enjoyed an odd mini vacation – a King-Kubrick-Nicholson The Shining hotel bar, a 1940s retro mineral bath and massage, elegant Italian restaurant server with a southern twang, 200 alligators at a petting zoo. Then we took a curiosity induced drive through Branson, Missouri – plastic fantastic, giant plastic King Kong, plastic Titanic iceberg, plastic chickens, and dead entertainers live in concert. Were we getting back to normal?

I still woke feeling as if I were being strangled, but only because I have high expectations. I had some energy, I slept hard, I worked and wrote and hiked. And I was asking myself non-cancer related questions suitable for a language nerd. Why do people redundantly say "the reason why" instead of "the reason?" And why have we gone from saying "we have to" to "we've got to"? And should that question mark go inside the quotation mark or outside, as if I were living in Great Britain or Spain? Are these questions that only plague writers? Or "older" writers? Or anyone obsessed with language?

Mid-November, I let my expectations overrun reality again. This was not the Hawaiian beach I'd envisioned. Eating was a chore and I couldn't find anything funny about my head being a bowling ball. And I felt too much empathy when I learned of a neighbors' new grandbaby being born with Downs Syndrome. I did "normal things" to distract myself and gutted it through. I would be 59 in a month, and would have to work until I was 70 or so, ten short years. But I was determined to climb mountains with my son and daughter, finish a cancer comedy, float the Eleven Point River, fly to Hawaii and Spain, and continually fight the inevitable slide into my parents' old age. "Rage, Rage Against the Dying of the Light."

My brother John, his son Brian, and I hiked a path winding through the hardwood forest at LaBarque Creek Conservation Area. On the way back, we discovered a new Conservation Area with a lake in the woods, drank a beer there, and I felt good. Maybe my life was starting to mirror "normalcy," with good days and bad. You know. Like most people?

November 22 came and went and nothing horrible happened, and I was on my way to being free. Shannon Nana readjusted my expectations like a chiropractor. We hugged goodbye. I imagined Kim and I visiting her someday on her island paradise. Then I drove to my parents house in Belleville and helped my Dad put up his Christmas lights.

On December 18, I entered another space capsule for a PET scan. As an experienced astronaut, I blasted off into chilly space, and landed casually. Until of course the next morning when I anticipated the results with only a little less panic than the last scan. At least this time, we got them early.

On December 20, I sent an email with the subject line "A Good PET."

"So my last follow-up scan, a PET scan, had some very interesting results. Perfect as a purring cat! Checked it twice and can't find anything that even remotely resembles cancer. So now I just have to continue healing and continue seeking that ever elusive normalcy."

My brother Jim responded, "This is wonderful news that made me very happy."

His wife Kathi wrote, "Your good test results are absolutely outstanding to hear about. What a difficult year it's been for you and Kim. 2013 will be much better."

Eric texted, "Thank God. That is fantastic. I love you brother."

I talked to my brother John. "That's great," he said, and we discussed our next hike, perhaps to Lower Rock Creek.

My Denver no-good-brother-in-law John texted, "That's awesome news. Knew all along you'd make it! Merry Xmas and count your blessings you won't have to put up with me this holiday season!"

John Reichle expressed his steady support, much in the same way he steadfastly carried gear up the mountain slope in the Wind River Range and managed the emotions of Metropolitan students. Andi showered her usual surge of uplifting words. I heard from everyone who knew the deal, Metropolitan math teacher Bob Johnson, former St. Louis Writers Guild president Robin Theiss, Beth, her husband Brad, my cousin Linda....

Claire texted, "Great news! Are you doing something stupid to celebrate?"

Lisa emailed, "Your news is the BEST holiday gift one could pray for. Love to Kim, and best wishes to you all for a wonderful holiday."

Ken Yorgan responded, "Way to go, you lucky bastard! What a fuckin' ride, eh? I'm happy for you, man, I really am. Now get back to work."

Lin Shook emailed, "So does that mean you'll be having a 'run naked in the snow' party for your birthday? Let me know and I'll get a mega-bus ticket."

Julie texted, "Yay! What a freakin' year! Jeff that is very good. I'm so thrilled that you're OK (and that I was right: you'll be fine:)"

John Zavgren emailed, "Jeff: That's GREAT news! I'm SO happy to hear that you're out of the woods. What a weird twisted stressful year... But, I have some bad news for you. You will never be normal. Never."

I responded, "Thanks for reminding me why we're friends."

And so on I was reminded of family and friends and the sheer joy of being alive.

I got an email from Christian Bone, someone I have never met, who I've only known through email, who nonetheless was a survivor and prayed for me. "That's great news. Any time you're battling cancer it's a weird year." Then he described his four day wait for results, being told they were "abnormal" and waiting another eight days for the doctor visit. But "all was well. Thanks for sharing your good news."

I responded, "That must have driven you nuts. I would have been jumping out of my skin."

And then it occurred to me. Only then? I should pray for him. So I did, at least a few lines anyway. I'll throw one in each time I think of him. No one will ever be sure if it does any good, but at some point, all you have left is faith. An internet article caught me off guard. I read that all cancer patients believe they are going to survive. That in itself isn't very comforting, doesn't do much for my own belief. Obviously, many of them die anyway. So it could happen to me, and Christian Bone, and anyone, even with prayer.

I was reminded of something Christian emailed earlier in this process. "I've gone through my battles with cancer and I'll never forget them but the sharp edges of those memories get smoother all the time."

Yes, the edges are getting smoother for me, but it doesn't take much for your faith to be shaken. I had heard

Doctor Gay say that the PET would be the "last scan." Possibly he said "for a while." But in my everlasting attempt to use my imagination to manipulate reality, I believed that I was "home free." Kim of course had known better and tried to tell me. I interpreted that last scan to mean last doctor appointment, last everything, and that maybe in a year or so, I'd have to visit.

On January 3, 2013, almost a year since my first surgery, and a few days before I would return to teaching, we went to the PET follow up appointment. A rotating shift resident came into the office first. My doppelganger was long gone. This new guy reminded me a little of Doctor Fred.

I deviated from my tightrope walk of wanting to know and not wanting to know. I asked this Doctor Fred incarnate why, since the scan was clean, did I need to come to these follow-ups. "Why?"

Now I'm asking myself why I asked the question. His answer was straightforward enough and confirmed what Kim was trying to tell me. If the big C is going to come back, it will most likely happen in three to five years.

"What's the point?" I asked, "There's nothing we can do about it anyway."

"Well," he said and I expected him to add, Mr. May, like Doctor Fred, "We wouldn't have you come in if there was nothing we could do. Hopefully, we would catch it early."

"Then what?"

"We could do surgery. Maybe a little targeted radiation if it comes back in a spot that hasn't been radiated before."

Doctor Haughey said radiation was a "one-time shot." Who was this guy to say any different? And Doctor Gay had said at one point, "We have to think we hit a home run here." And my radiation side effects were going away, my ulcerations diminished, felt like they were almost gone.

"Okay," I said. "But I'm still not sure why I have to keep coming back here."

"Well, we also check for radiation side-effects, just to see how you're doing, see if you've developed any sores or anything."

"I'm fine, I'm in great shape."

He agreed, and I thought this guy didn't know me. Doctor Gay came in and we had our usual laid back pleasant conversation, and he confirmed what the resident said, that there will be frequent doctor visits for the next three to five years, the next appointment with him in three months. He said that he didn't see the need for more scans, just make sure that I had a follow up with Doctor Haughey.

So I went in thinking I was home free and came out praying to God to spare me. What would happen if they cut my tongue again? The thought was too horrible to think about, and again had me on my knees. Dear God!

Does belief then require purposely avoiding knowing? If I had avoided knowing about the three to five years and the probabilities, would I be better off? Or would that be like not knowing about global climate change until your house was on fire or submerged? I read that 2012 was the hottest year on record for the lower forty-eight, that one record after another was falling. What about 2013? (Probably you are reading this after the summer of '13. What was it like?)

I had trouble with "probability." Did that mean my cancer would "probably" come back in three to five? Would the fear and doubt ever go away? Three to five years of doctor visits, any one of which might have some resident say, "Interesting."

When I see Doctor Haughey, I won't ask. Don't want to ask. No need to imagine the worst. I had lost my balance, fallen off my tightrope, and the fall didn't feel too good.

So I must force an end to this hilarious Cancer Comedy. My full recovery as elusive as my comedy as I grapple with "long-term" radiation side effects, lingering dry mouth, lack of taste, and other "things." Maybe psychological. Will I grapple with them for the rest of my life? Sometimes, it seems I will be in eternal recovery.

But I vow, now and forever, that I will never stop, I will always seek my elusive full recovery, and I will enjoy the effort as I age, enjoy the love I remember, the love I have, and the love yet to come. I can do all of this only because of the skill of a great surgeon, the right attitude, and the love and support of family and friends. Without that, I might not be writing this now, at this glorious moment.

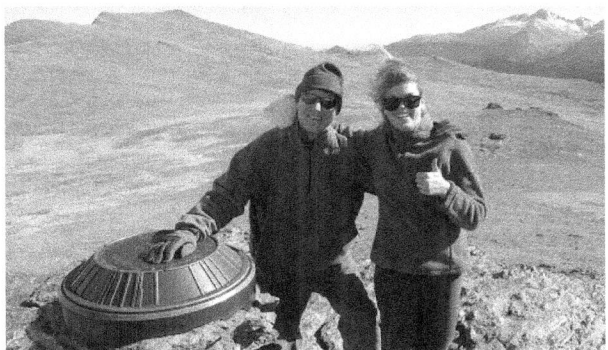

Update: Life Is Good

Introduction

So all I really wanted to do was update the cover, with my full name and so on and I had it ready to go in 2021...but reality seldom seems to match our intentions...

If you are reading this, then you might be wondering if I have "fully recovered." The short answer is no. But darn close, close enough to live fully, both fun times and some not-so-much. And my sense of humor has been severely tested again. Ha. Ha.

Doctor Haughey, the surgeon who saved my life, moved to Florida and was replaced by a young oncologist, Doctor Ryan Jackson. During one of my yearly scope-up-the-nose examinations, I panicked about what turned out to be a cold sore under my tongue. Doctor Jackson shrugged off my concern and said, "You're cured."

So why endure the yearly dread, the visits to his eleventh floor office, the parking garage, traffic, city noise, and the fear that "they" just might find something? I didn't go back. Until I had to.

Part I – Recovery

In 2013, I returned to work as an English Composition instructor, and found it difficult to enunciate some letter combinations, especially words requiring volume and emphasis. And with reduced spittle control, I didn't dare lecture too close to a student. Drinking seemed to loosen my mangled tongue a bit, but teaching while drunk didn't seem like a good idea.

That first post-cancer summer included the Chicago Art Institute, backpacking with my daughter Sarah in Rocky Mountain National Park, fishing with my brother Jim in Wyoming, and an Ozark float trip – a year of healthy physical activity.

I developed a thought-trick for overcoming the feeling of perpetual strangulation. As each moment unfolded, I lived as fully as possible, and then immediately after, recalled the moment, omitting the "discomfort." After awhile I couldn't remember which events occurred before and which after.

In 2014, Kim and I drove through the Deep South, the Shiloh Civil War battlefield, swam in the gulf, visiting our friends Julie and her husband Daryl who had relocated to Alabama for a new job. You will recall Julie as a consistent force for optimism, often telling me, "You'll be fine Jeff." We visited Sarah in Denver, camped in the mountains next to roaring white water with Lin Shook, Lynn Wakefield and her brother, taking day hikes into the wilderness. Our minister-sex-therapist friend Bob passed away and we sprinkled his ashes in the Eleven Point River, floating, swimming, camping, and diving into icy cold Ozark springs.

On November 9, at my Dad's request, I went to check on my little brother Eric. His front door was locked, his dog barking and whimpering inside. I broke in through the window and found him in bed, his body stiff, fingers crooked, blank eyes staring at his dirty ceiling, years of too much alcohol. Clearly, he was not merely sleeping in.

My brother John and I made the always charming, onerous hour drive into the Illinois flatlands of Belleville to tell our parents. My Mom, arms folded and head down on the kitchen table, kept repeating, "Walter is Eric dead?" Her refrain became my ear worm, sometimes accompanied by the 1975 Electric Light Orchestra, "Can't get it out of my head," and occasionally superimposed with 1965 Little Anthony and the Imperials "Going out of my head, day and night, night and day."

Early in 2015, Dad needed dialysis and Mom's dementia worsened; she told a story and laughed and everybody laughed along with her, and two minutes later she would tell the same story and laugh, and again we laughed along with her. Shortly after Mom passed away at 95, Dad told me how he'd sat next to her, both in wheelchairs, and asked her for "one last kiss." He got nothing, so he asked again, and again nothing, but on the third request… "She gave me the biggest kiss you could imagine."

That summer, I wrote a novella, *Margery*, about an introverted backpacker wandering off trail and discovering an otherworldly town nestled in a mountain basin where, as one reviewer stated, "the transition between life and death is defined by each individual with the help of hallucinogenic mushrooms." *Margery* was a finalist for Homebound Publications 2022 Landmark Prize and was published May 2023 by Paper Angel Press.

Dad died in February 2016, at 96, and his last words to me, a week before his passing, were a gift: "Life is good." And I find it "funny" that this book is framed by that cliché.

Kim and I took a 3,000 mile road trip west in my manual transmission Mazda 3, visiting Kim's brother in Fort Worth, then San Antonio and the Alamo. One of the scariest movie scenes I can remember was Jim Bowie with his famous knife slicing at bayonets, only Bowie and the bayonets are shown. (Dying in battle was a consistent childhood theme for me and my brothers.) In the movie Bowie had been courageously wounded but in reality he had advanced tuberculosis.

We drove across the west Texas desert to Guadalupe National Park to hike the highest point. But it was on fire. So we spent the night in Roswell looking for aliens, and then on to the highest point in New Mexico. But it was buried in snow. "Some say the world will end in fire / Some say in ice."

In 2017, we became all-inclusive resort people on the Mexican Rivera, and visited the ruins at Tulum. My daughter and I backpacked Segment 10 of the Colorado Trial and climbed Mount Massive. Near the summit we met a guy recovering from lymphoma and exchanged teary eyed encouragement and congratulations.

In 2018, we travelled to Costa Rica, zip-lines, iguana, crocodiles, booze, and sunsets. Then my oldest brother, John, scared the hell out of us with a near fatal heart attack and my neck started bothering me, seemingly more than usual, a tightness that wouldn't leave me alone. So I did what I've always done and tried to write my way out of it, resulting in a semi-autobiographical novel – *The Blue Ink Notes*. In it, the unreliable narrator moves to a small run-down house in the Ozark woods where he decides to write the perfect suicide note (another impossible quest). The result is a darkly humorous, hopeful narrative. (Still unpublished as of Fall 2023.)

We visited Kim's sister Beth in Maine, sailed, hiked, fished and of course ate lobster. After that, I organized a Glacier National Park trip with old Metropolitan School colleagues, including John Reichle and Andi Boyd and a former student, to hike on glaciers before they melted away. Unfortunately, we had to maneuver over 150 trees, give or take a few, felled by a recent storm and had to turn back, climbing over them a second time, settling for fantastic views, the receding glaciers forever just beyond our grasp.

In 2019, my heart-attack oldest-brother John suffered through his wife passing away from urinary tract cancer. So what else could he do but join me in a classic American Road Trip? We blundered along back roads, historic sites and natural wonders, fishing with our brother Jim in Wyoming, then on to a friend's ranch near Saratoga. I left John there and headed to Denver where my daughter and I climbed Mt. Elbert, the highest point in Colorado. While we were basking in our summit success, John called and told me that Jim and his wife Kathi rolled their truck in the backcountry. Both nearly died. What a buzz kill. It seemed my brothers, Eric, John, and now Jim – those bastards were retaliating just because I scared them with a gruesome cancer.

After John and I visited Jim and Kathi in separate hospitals, we reconnected in Ft. Collins and started our backroad journey home, stopping to "climb" the highest point in Kansas, Mt. Sunflower, summit temperature 101.

By the time the superbly dystopian year 2020 came along, our children were heavily into drugs and alcohol – that was our standard joke. Sarah was earning promotions in the marijuana industry and Sam was enthusiastic about the future while working at a brewery in St. Louis. But of course everything changed. And that of course is an understatement.

Around spring break, classes transitioned online and since I hated teaching online, it was easy for me to officially retire.

Dental issues appeared early in 2020, and one evening when nerves were zinging across my chin, I fell onto the carpet as if bombs were exploding over my head. (The term PTSD seems overused – how could it possibly compare to my Dad's war trauma?) After a Xanax, the panic subsided. Now I smile and show off my implants and caps and exorbitant dental bills.

A therapist asked why my ghoulish radiation mask was, after ten years, still residing in a dark corner of the basement. Good question. So I tried to give it away, but couldn't find anyone who wanted it, not even an artist. That Halloween, I positioned my mask in the trash can so that it stared up at the trash man. Hope he had a sense of humor.

Kim and I rented a car and took a carefully-planned, Covid-aware summer road trip. By turning onto remote gravel roads, we easily avoided gas station bathrooms. We entered hotel rooms with disinfectant, used our own pillows and sheets on top of theirs, and left everything cleaner than when we arrived. At the time, the Great Plains had very few Covid cases, so we drove to Hawkeye Point, the highest point in Iowa. In North Dakota, we hiked the four mile round trip to the highpoint, White Butte. In nearby Bowman, we walked down main street and saw only one person, a guy lounging in front of a bar, dirty jeans and long sleeve shirt, cigarette dangling, legs crossed, eyes closed, who suddenly sat up straight and asked, "How do you cook a Panda?" We didn't know. "In a pan, duh." Now we know.

In Wyoming Jim and his wife had more or less recovered from their near fatal accident, and we went fishing with them in the high country. Then to Montrose and my cousin Christy and her spouse and a daytrip to the Black Canyon of the Gunnison, sheer cliffs of striated metamorphic granite, the Gunnison River snaking through the canyon. And no trip west is complete without seeing Sarah in Denver, this time rock climbing with her current partner, Bryan. We took the back roads home, avoiding the misleading arrows and interstate spaghetti of Kansas City.

Unfortunately, problems with Kim's dad were mounting and, as the oldest and the only sibling in St. Louis, taking care of him became mostly her responsibility, which naturally included me. In October my neck suddenly swelled and burst open with a lymph node infection. My primary care nurse confirmed the infection but also said, "I want you to see your oncologist." That perfectly logical suggestion almost knocked me to the floor.

The infection healed and a November trip to the oncologist and an ultrasound showed "lymph nodes demonstrate normal morphology." Kim set up lymphedema treatment. The specialists were outstanding and I felt better by the time treatment ended.

While people argue about everything, including when a decade begins and ends, to me 2020 felt like the end. We were passing into a new decade, stunned by the pandemic, and overcome by crises…political, cultural, climate.

Part II – Fighting a Fistula?

For us and perhaps many of you, 2021 was even more challenging. In the first few months, I worked hard helping Kim sell off and reinvest some of her Dad's real estate holdings. And we were optimistic about driving an hour and a half to Rolla for our first dose of the vaccine.

However, the ghost of Nurse April finally caught up with me. Near the first day of that cruelest month, my neck swelled much worse than before and started leaking various colored fluids, then broke open to a monstrous, gaping quarter-sized hole, perfect for electrical amplification.

It looked on its way toward a peaceful resolution when we took a second vaccine trip to Rolla and visited "Uranus Fudge Factory, where the best fudge comes from Uranus." But my primary care doctor sent me back to the oncologist because they were concerned "about tracks that could be holding infection in the node or neck and cause recurrent episodes." With Kim increasingly entangled with her Dad, I went alone into the city to see Doctor Jackson's assistant, Melissa.

After a CT scan, Melissa said a biopsy was needed because they "saw something" on the scan and it looked "big" and "significant." When I asked for reassurance, suggesting that it could still just be an infection, she didn't want to give "false hope." I asked again, and again she said "false hope." Nice. I needed to find some magic mushrooms and start planning my funeral.

The next day they stabbed me in the neck five times trying to get a good "ultrasound-guided fine needle aspiration." The biopsy report appeared online clearly stating "negative for malignancy" and "mixed inflammation and reactive changes." Kim asked, "Does this mean Jeff does *not* have cancer?" Melissa responded, "No cancer, just scar-tissue."

Things were going along swimmingly and it had healed up almost entirely by April 30. Unfortunately, on May first it turned dark and swollen, broke open and created another hole, a recurring pattern of optimism and setback, hope and "oh hell" lasting around 18 months. Many times, during this cycle of healing and desperation, I had to use a stick (usually made by taking the cotton off a Q-tip) and stuff gauze strips about a quarter inch deep into my neck, often screaming to comfort the process. (Contact me if you want a detailed description and gross pictures.)

On May 13, we went to see Doctor Jackson and his assistant Lisa Shoemaker at the West County Barnes location, much closer and easier for us. Also right next to where I got all that lovely radiation ten years ago. Doctor Jackson injected silver nitrate. His notes posted online read "No fistula seen. Discussed that I hope this resolves spontaneously. Surgery would be quite extensive." The silver nitrate provided colorful skin changes, but did nothing to stop the wound cycle.

On May 25, we went to Barnes Radiology for a swallow test. The radiologist had been enticed out of retirement because of the pandemic. We shared the standard joke: Radiation is the gift that keeps on giving. He talked amiably about his son's stem cell research and how radiation would one day be considered barbaric.

A few days later, the report read: "No evidence of fistulization... does not appear to track all the way to the skin." However, the fluids coming out my neck were looking even more suspiciously like my smoothies. West County Lisa agreed that while extremely small, it must be a fistula. My standard joke, repeated way too often and for too long – I could tap my neck and drink my beer twice. Great value!

On June 5, Kim and I drove to Galena and hiked the highpoint in Illinois, staying at a lodge overlooking the Mississippi, drinking, eating edibles, "letting loose" like a notorious couple just released from jail. The blood and saliva leaking down my neck didn't interfere with our fun.

On June 10, we went to Barnes West expecting to discuss fistula treatment, but Doctor Jackson said, "Who said it was a fistula?" Truly a WTF moment. He attributed the strange color of my discharge to the silver nitrate. We left hoping that it would heal on its own. The online notes provided a smattering of clarity: "Barium swallow did not show fistula. If persistent will consider removal and reconstruction." Removal of what? And reconstruction...like after the Civil War?

In July, we visited Ken Yorgan and his new wife Sue in Racine, then the bizarre House on the Rock, the Wisconsin highpoint, the Minnesota highpoint, Cliff Dweller hotel on Lake Superior, and the source of the Mississippi with lots of people splashing around turning the pristine water brown.

However, the discharge was still matching my meals, particularly green spinach. On August 15, at 9 pm, I was "fed up" so I did a home "lab test." I held water with red food coloring in my mouth. Soon, the red water bubbled and flowed down my neck.

On August 26, I told Doctor Jackson about my home test and showed him pictures. He said, "Sorry you had to endure this for so long." Now, he said, it was reasonable to try a surgical correction, "a wide local excision of the granulation tract and local adjacent tissue transfers... with multiple layer closure... has a fair chance of healing his wound." Not good, or very good, or excellent. But fair is fair enough. We appreciated starting out small. If this "correction" didn't work, then "we always have the big surgery." Seven days in the hospital and a month with feeding tube through the nose. Last time, if you'll recall, my nose took some abuse. Would I finally end up like one of those poor souls at MD Anderson with chunks of their face missing?

Because second and third and fourth opinions had led us to Doctor Haughy who saved my life, I thought it prudent to see at least one other oncologist. On September 23, Kim and I went to see Doctor James Boyd at Mercy. From the moment we met him in his office, it seemed clear he was determined to find cancer. He said in his 30 years, he hadn't seen this happen so long after treatment, and we had to find out why it was happening, and he was ordering a PET scan to see if anything "lit up" and, by the way, "cancer treatment has come a long way in ten years."

My cousin Christy arrived a few hours after my engaging pep talk with Doctor Boyd, and we began the process of moving our 94-year old aunt out of her Belleville condo and into an Assisted Living facility. For a week, we helped her move. During this time, the PET scan results came back inconclusive, couldn't determine if it was malignancy or inflammation.

Two days later, Doctor Boyd decided at 10:15 PM to amend the test result with his own note, which I read around 11 PM on September 30. "Appears to be likely positive for recurrence." Huh? What the hell did "appears to be likely positive" mean? On the bright side, the PET scan didn't "light up" anywhere else. But how do you cope with "appears likely?" The perpetual choke hold on my neck tightened. I immediately scheduled outpatient surgery with Doctor Jackson.

On October 21, Kim and I walked into the same hospital entrance as ten years ago, past all those interesting memories, past where I had wheeled my IV outside, head wrapped in bandages, breathing in the city air and longing for escape.

The surgery went well. Doctor Jackson didn't see any evidence of cancer, but would send it off for a biopsy, a standard procedure. A few days later, the test result was posted online but I was reluctant to look at it. Who knows what kind of "appears-likely" note might be attached. Then the stitches separated and the gaping hole in my neck returned. Immediately, I emailed Lisa. She called early the next morning, asking questions, wanting me to send a photo. "But," I said, "There's no cancer, right?"

The biopsy was negative, no effing cancer. Lisa emailed instructions to soak gauze in prescription saline-solution, pack the hole three times a day, and we would see Doctor Jackson on the follow up appointment November 11, Veteran's day. (Okay Dad, am I a veteran of sorts now? No, I'll never match your service to country and freedom, but you remain an inspiration.) Three times a day, I stuffed saline dampened gauze into my neck.

On our Veteran's Day visit, Kim talked about the stitches not holding, but Doctor Jackson said it was because of the over-radiated skin. He suggested that the radiation protocol should be changed. (Obviously every case is different, but if you are facing radiation, you might want to ask incisive questions. Do I really need it? What level? Is it too much?) After pulling off my bandage, Doctor Jackson became enthusiastic, even using the word "awesome," and we cracked a few dumb jokes and we left his office feeling very good.

A couple days later I read the online notes, "Mr. May returns with his spouse." (How often have I "returned" with Kim?) "He is doing excellent after closure of his oral cutaneous fistula…no drainage whatsoever as far as saliva or liquids…healing extremely well…. I will see him in one month or sooner if issues arise. Likely this will be completely healed at that point." (Did the doctor finally believe me? It *was* a fistula.)

After a few days, however, the long slog of healing became apparent. Three times, every day, the dreaded bandage change, morbid fantasies of foul exorcist stench squirting out my neck, and I cringed while treating my wound, ritualistically following instructions, wash hands, prepare gauze, push it in as far as I could using my stick, my bathroom sink a surgeon's table.

After several weeks of agonizingly slow healing, I ate a big spinach salad for dinner and that night a discharge on the gauze looked suspiciously green. I was convinced that the fistula had returned, emailing Lisa, with pictures. "Apologize for being a bother again..."

Before the end of the day, a response: "Dr. Jackson thinks 'it looks fantastic actually...things look good and would not change anything at this time.' He did not think the drainage was related to the salad."

So for the next eight days I changed my dressing three times a day as quickly as possible while avoiding looking at it for more than a split second. No more obsessive self-examination with photographs.

At our next appointment, Doctor Jackson was clearly pleased, and so were we, the mood jovial. He said the wound was almost healed, and I could just use a Band-Aide and a little antibiotic and we would see each other again in about six months. However, having seen it *almost* heal about "eight billion" times, only to swell and burst open again, I remained wary.

Very tentatively, cautiously, Kim and I started talking about Hawaii, that last state we both have never been to, and were planning on visiting ten years ago when this little cancer comedy interfered.

But on Christmas Eve morning, my wound was on the verge of catastrophe again, and Kim and I got a call from her Dad's caregiver. By the time we got to his house, he was gone. We spent the next four hours with the necessary paperwork and waiting for the body to be removed. That night, my wound was leaking food and saliva. I would be fighting a fistula forever, nothing good about it except that pithy bit of alliteration. In a weird, perverse way, I was relieved because all along, I was plagued with nagging doubts about the surgery. Wonderful to be proven right, isn't it?

After another email exchange with Doctor Jackson's nurse Lisa, in which I expressed my desire to avoid the hospital during the current Covid surge, and suggested vacuum therapy and super glue, she responded that I would be their priority in the New Year and would "set you up with something called a wound vac." The obvious joke: would they use a Hoover?

On a positive note, I found that Walgreens Hydrocolloid Gel Bandages combined with a small ball of gauze would hold back the fluid for at least 24 hours and didn't irritate the surrounding skin too much. With such a method, I could conceivably backpack into the mountains.

Part III – Radiation Resolution

I entered the New Year 2022 enthusiastic about Hydrocolloid Gel Bandages. While sorting through the fallout of my father-in-law's passing, we listened to the wound center expert repeat familiar BS: when we see you next it should be healed completely. But of course that didn't happen, and we went back to Dr. Jackson and scheduled a March 11 surgery, "only a half-hour and a few stitches." Kim needed to be with our daughter in Denver so Dave Lancaster filled in.

Naturally the unexpected occurred again and the minor surgery turned into two hours, and I came out of it barely coherent, babbling about going hiking and drinking beer.

Sam came over and spent the night but had to leave in the morning. Our next door neighbor brought me a smoothie and I told her I was fine, but in reality could barely function, setting the smoothie on the fireplace hearth but missing and spilling it all over our Oriental rug, the rug having its own story from when Kim found it 40 years ago.

Once again, after surgery, the stiches stretched out exposing another hole, and I was convinced it didn't work. My mood was terrible and I responded to Kim and others with a fuck here and a fuck there, everywhere a fuck.

When we visited Doctor Jackson on the May 31, my mood wasn't any better, but he was encouraging and empathetic, and said that this was "only" the second surgery, and so far we'd managed to avoid the week in the hospital with skin grafts and tubes and everything else unpleasant.

During this time, I taught Fiction writing classes, barely able to manage it, often chasing hydrocodone with beer, but those cheerful adult students seemed to enjoy themselves.

Meanwhile, my father-in-law's body was barely stiff when Kim's siblings started fighting. In April of 2022, her sister Beth turned over the Trusteeship to Kim, and our previous work load doubled, working hard from morning until night almost every day, gathering paperwork, communication with lawyers, banks, brokers, and doing the extraordinarily demanding work of cleaning out her childhood home, a place where her parents spent 56 years and her Dad had a hard time throwing things away – Rx bottles, screws, lawn mowers, broken furniture and so on. It remains a darkly humorous story too detailed to include in this update, except to say that after toil and frustration, coinciding with my radiation wound struggles we finally settled their family's Trust. But as a result, we lost the friendship of two siblings. It's almost as if they passed away. (Curiously enough, we've remained friends with Anne and her husband John.)

My neck didn't feel too good lugging heavy items all day every day, but the work was necessary, the right thing to do, so we trudged on. On the bright side, the main hole healed up again. No discharge! Doctor Jackson had put me on 500 mg Cephalexin four times a day.

However, after a three mile hike at a conservation area, I wondered why my car smelled like horse manure long after passing the horse stables. My bandage and neck-gaiter were soaked. Right above the main hole, close to the jaw, swelled up to the size of a golf ball with two pin-sized discharge bubbles.

April first came and went, the anniversary of horrible events, and now it all seemed like a whack-a-mole game, the main hole healed only to have this new one bulge out and announce its presence, a blister-like swelling, bursting and repeating. However, the swelling eventually went down and the discharge stopped.

Feeling very optimistic going into the appointment on May 12, 2022 with no bandage on my neck for the first time in over a year, I thought we would all sit in his office, have a laugh, and the doctor would send me on my way "cured."

Close but no cigar and I didn't dare ask him about the cigars my brother John made me smoke while out fishing. Doctor Jackson cheerfully explained what happened with the surgery. He claimed again it was not a fistula, solely the result of too much radiation. Apparently, during the surgery, he found one tract all the way to the hyoid bone. That hell-fire radiation had affected the hyoid bone, necrosis, and a piece had rotted off and had tried to make its way through the skin. He had gone in and shaved the bone down. (Well, blow me down!)

So, I thought, all good, why is he crossing his fingers again hoping it all works. He put me on a regimen of medication for the next three months to help heal the bone. The obvious supposition, which I didn't dare ask about, was that it could happen again if the bone decided to flake off again and then I would end up being even flakier than before. See how easy it is to find humor. Ha. Ha.

The medication routine was sort of "funny," Vitamin E daily, red one twice daily Monday through Friday with food, white Saturday and Sunday with food, big red oval Saturday and Sunday with or without food and small white only on Saturday on an empty stomach with 8 ounces of water and stay upright for 30 minutes. What sort of toil and trouble bat crap crazy stew was this?

We had about two months of no bandage and everything was looking good – aside from the panic, anxiety, extreme tightness, the feeling of being at the end of a barbed wire noose and dancing desperately on a wobbly chair.

In defiance probably, Kim and I took a trip to door county, Wisconsin for a few days. Driving was tough. I was miserable, the tightness and burning, the fear of being forever "uncomfortable." Kim told me that my bone could be deteriorating and it might have to be replaced. How comforting. On occasion, my wife was a double-edged sword of information.

Saturday, June 25, 2022, I was miserable and terrified, and emailed Lisa Shoemaker the following, "Will try calling you Monday morning. I don't understand why my neck feels worse than when I had the hole. Is this part of the normal healing process? Or is something wrong?"

Doctor Jackson ordered hyperbaric chamber treatment. At first, I though great, did it before, around 2014, being ultra-cautious before a tooth extraction, and it was a breeze. This time however it became a torture chamber, something my brother John referred to as my spa treatment. And yes, celebrities believe it can make you look and feel younger. However, for me, every morning at 7 AM, the ninety minute sessions sealed in a tube, 40 sessions consuming my summer, felt nothing like a relaxing spa. It required Xanax and Ambien to endure. And then! After my very last treatment! A pin hole of leaking fluids appeared. The path to the hyoid bone was healed, but this was a new and different path, one not yet taken.

Two days after my release from the hyper-torture chamber, I forged my own trail and took a trip – a trip treatment with psilocybin therapy. Contrary to what I may have implied, this was my first time using hallucinogenic drugs. Did it help? Hard to say, but it didn't hurt. I laughed for the first hour and a half, lying down with eyes covered and hallucinations bouncing around the inside of my eyelids, a roller coaster ride through my mind. No new revelations, but perhaps a deeper appreciation of them. Intermittently during the trip, I was fighting off attempts to butcher my neck.

I contacted Lisa again – nicely communicating something like, what the hell do we do now? "This is a very complex case," she said. How would the big surgery work when nobody knew where the hole on the inside was? "I don't think he ever knew where it originated."

My choices were to take antibiotics long term or go for the surgery without him knowing where to go. I asked what "long term" meant. And heard a familiar phrase. "For the rest of your life." Well, okay, how long would that be?

Kim was continually researching fistulas. She found an obscure study about a woman who had gotten drunk, fallen, and accidentally stabbed a broken beer bottle into her neck, and subsequently developed a fistula. The doctors treated it with a scopolamine patch. After three days, the fistula was gone, the patch diminished saliva in the tract allowing it to dry out and heal.

On our wedding anniversary October 24, 2022, I got an email. "Here is what he said about the big surgery and fistula. 'I am still not convinced he has a leak. Maybe keep him on suppressive Keflex' which we are doing already. I know that you disagree about the leak. He actually recommends after a week or so switching the Keflex to just once a day, instead of four. I will ask him about the scopolamine patch and get back to you."

The Doctor prescribed eight scopolamine patches. After using one, I could tell the difference. There was no tell-tale tiny bubble on the wound. Even so, I remained cautious, and used several more patches, and over a couple months eased off the antibiotics, titrating down to three, two, and… then there were none.

There was no hole, no wound, no sign of infection. It appeared my wife had once again sustained me with her life-saving research. While still struggling with the barbed wire noose, at least it was healed over. At least I looked good enough and good enough is enough to fool others into thinking I was just fine.

Now it was Kim's turn, a melanoma on her baby toe, the roles reversing, waiting for her tests to show that it hadn't spread, scheduling surgery, healing, a moment when she panicked, "It's not working." I tried hard to match her support during my travails, providing reassurance, helping with difficult decisions. Aside from having to do some mental gymnastics, she is okay, fantastic, not even a single sign of melanoma, although she does have to go in every few months, just to make sure.

The End of an Update

While not technically showing signs of lymphedema (no swelling), I continued treatment well into 2023 because it helped with the tightness and neuropathy, a word I'd been trying to avoid. Treatment is tricky, and the diagnosis comes with dire prognostications. However, I talked to a psychiatrist and we settled on trying 25mg of amitriptyline to help with the burning.

In March, we went to Bentonville, Arkansas, on to Mount Magazine lodge, hiking to the highpoint. Several moments were amusing, but the drive home was difficult, my neck burning with the intensity of a year's worth of panic. We upped the Amitriptyline to 50mg.

In early April, we drove to visit our daughter in Idaho Springs, Colorado, then on to Pikes Peak, and Oklahoma's highest point, Black Mesa. My neck was bothersome but not brutal, and I had rediscovered a capacity for fun. My trick for living life and omitting the memories of discomfort was beginning to work again, although not nearly as easily.

During May and June, we exchanged emails with my cousins, Ruth and Sarah, who live next to the village of Volcano. We have plane tickets, resort reservations, and the resolve for a September visit the Big Island, Oahu, and Kauai, a far west trip over ten years in the making.

In July, we took a little "in-between trip" to South Dakota, over 2000 miles in five days, the usually clear western plains cloaked in haze and smoke from Canadian wildfires, and I hiked to the highpoint, Black Elk Peak (formerly Harney Peak). Lots of hikers scrambled past Native American prayer flags to play on the expansive boulders. Kim and I skipped Rushmore (been there before) and opted to visit the Crazy Horse Memorial, years ago barely recognizable, now a clear face and hand carved into the rock, and a very large tourist center. In fact the whole Black Hills area was swarming with tourists, (making the trip to Black Mesa, Oklahoma seem luxuriously exclusive). We drove the back roads home, spending the night in Broken Bow, Nebraska, and Chillicothe, Missouri.

This "update" has gone on way too long. My neck is well enough for me to bring this to a conclusion. If I tried to include everything, it might become an autobiography, and no one in their right mind would want that. So it must end. I'm not going to be writing from the grave. If there is an afterlife, hope it's not this warm. (Or like summers yet to arrive?)

Even though I still hike, bike, walk at least 20 miles a week, I am, like everyone else, getting older. Funny how that works. In fact, I might be old now. My seventieth birthday is waiting for me at the end of 2023.

Obviously, many suffer much worse than I do. Millions have succumbed to Covid-19. There's war in Ukraine, children slaughtered, the rights of women, genders, races… the looming climate catastrophe: fires, storms, flooding, searing heat waves across the globe, Earth's hottest recorded summer. Not a lot of humor in that is there? An impossible quest?

I have not given up, nor should you. In my own way, I pray for you and hope you've found something helpful in this update (at least the warning about radiation and the suggestion for fixing a fistula). If you are feeling downhearted, get up and move and keep moving. Even overly optimistic encouragement, bordering on lies, can be useful. Clichés and platitudes too, they are more useful than you might think and I willingly offer them to you. You're going to be okay. And that's no joke.

Hawaii is on the horizon.

Margery

As I hiked further into the woods, deeper than I'd ever gone before, I noticed darkness not only surrounding me from the thick canopy of hardwood trees, their leaves abnormally large, but also felt a heaviness in my heart, a tightness in my chest that was counter to all my previous experiences hiking into the wilderness.

Usually I felt exultant at the blood and oxygen and endorphins rushing through my body, making me thank God, nature, pure existence. But not this time as I forged along this narrow winding path, an innocent offshoot to the heavily used trail, a path that begged for exploring, one that reasonable people should be turning away from, but I've always felt drawn to the unknown, to the receding view around the bend. Sometimes I went too far, and this time I followed the path through underbrush, nothing more than the hint of a trail, and came upon a shallow clear stream about a dozen strides wide, roots of trees tangled along the banks.

I stopped and sat, backpack against a tree, my feet dangling from a root wad, feeling exhausted, almost crushed by the effort of moving. Not like me at all. What was going on? Should I sleep here, or retreat? Should I try to lay out my one-person tent along the small, twisting snake of a footpath and sleep? Darkness was seeping in around me and I suddenly felt more alone, more apprehensive than I had ever felt before.

ABOUT THE AUTHOR

Jeffrey Penn May has won several short fiction awards, received a Pushcart Prize nomination for his creative nonfiction and was a Landmark Prize finalist.

After earning his a B.A. in English and Psychology, a Masters in English Education, and a writer's certificate from the University of Missouri, Jeff worked as a waiter, hotel security officer, credit manager, deck hand, technical data engineer, principal of a small alternative school, and creative writing teacher.

Merging his writing with his outdoor adventures, Jeff has, among other things, floated a home-built raft from St. Louis to Memphis, navigated a John boat to New Orleans, dug for Pre-Columbian artifacts, and climbed mountains from Alaska to South America. In January, 2012, he was diagnosed with an extremely large and rare salivary gland tumor on the back of the tongue, throat and jaw, and is a cancer survivor.

Contact the author via www.askwritefish.com.

www.ingramcontent.com/pod-product-compliance
Lightning Source LLC
Chambersburg PA
CBHW070352290526
45790CB00004B/1455